The Prenatal Development of the Human Locomotor System

edited by
Jae Rhyong Yoon, M.D.

Professor Emeritus of Anatomy
Chonnam National University Medical School
Gwangju, Korea

Chonnam National University Press
Gwangju, Republic of Korea

Contributors

Baik Yoon Kim, M.D.
Emeritus Professor, Department of Anatomy
Chonnam National University Medical School
Gwangju, Korea

Choon Sang Bae, M.D.
Emeritus Professor, Department of Anatomy
Chonnam National University Medical School
Gwangju, Korea

Kyu Yoon Ahn, M.D.
Professor, Department of Anatomy
Chonnam National University Medical School
Gwangju, Korea

Kwang Il Nam, M.D.
Professor, Department of Anatomy
Chonnam National University Medical School
Gwangju, Korea

the Title of

The Prenatal Development of the Human Locomotor System

First published August 2019
Written by Jae Rhyong Yoon(M.D, Ph.D),
Chonnam National University
Publisher: Byung-Seok Jeong
ISBN 978-89-6849-651-6 (93510)
Price: 27,000 Won

Published by Chonnam National University Press,
77 Yongbong-ro, Bukgu, Gwangju,
Republic of Korea, 61186
Tel: 82-62-530-0571/3, Fax: 82-62-530-0579

Printed and bound in the Republic of Korea

CIP No : CIP2019032629

Preface

The knowledge of embryology is very significant in understanding of the function and structure of human bones and joints. In the whole human growth and development, the general form of human bone and joint in the early stage of the prenatal development was quite similar to that of the adult. Thus having a good grasp of the morphological development from the early embryonic stage to the full term should be greatly helpful for the understanding both normal structure and congenital malformation of the human body well. Recently due to the upgraded technological efficiency of diagnostic ultrasound and magnetic resonance imaging, the fetal period of human growth and development has risen as one intense field of academic investigation and scrutiny.

All samples in this book have been collected from human embryos and fetuses produced for the purpose of therapeutic abortion at the Department of Obstetrics and Gynecology in Chonnam National University Hospital. Most of the contents and the color photo-micrographs stem from my past researches conducted at the Department of Anatomy in Chonnam University Medical School for about thirty years. It is my greatest honor here that some pictures resulted from co-authored works with my splendid colleagues. Most research outcomes included in this book had been already publicized in a variety of academic journals.

Besides let me stress that for the estimation of embryonic developmental stages, Carnegie stage invented by Streeter, and later upgraded by O'Rahilly and Muller have been utilized. Fetal age has been estimated by menstrual age. Finally an estimation of crown-rump length have been based upon Choi's tables.

I sincerely hope that this book may help readers understand better the whole developmental process of human embryos and fetuses, as well as clinical importance of congenital malformation and pathological conditions as well.

Acknowledgement

First of all, let me express my heartfelt gratitude to my former colleagues in the Department of Anatomy of Chonnam University Medical School: Professors, Sung Sik Park, Baik Yoon Kim, Choon Sang Bae, Kyu Yoon Ahn, and Kwang Il Nam, who helped me with the informative advice and heartful cooperation. I wish to especially thank professor Jae Kwon Choi for the help, support, and encouragement of during the preparation of this book.

During the several years it took to elaborate this book, our many colleagues have kindly aided me in different ways, and I thank them very cordially. Without their help, this work would have remained only idea. I thank warmly my former technical assistance of the Department of Anatomy, Mrs. Jung Ja Chung and Mr. Chul Soo Ahn, for their tireless work in cutting and staining sections for photography.

Finally, I thank our families for the great patience and sympathy they have shown to me during the several years of preparation of the present work. If this book would be helpful to the researches of the readers, they should share credit.

Criteria for Estimating Developmental Stages in Human Embryos and Fetuses*

Stages	Crown-Rump Length (mm)	Age (weeks)	Main External Characteristics
13	6	4	Upper limb buds are flipper-like. Lower limb buds appear.
14	7	4.5	Upper limb buds are paddle-shaped.
15	8	4.5	Hand plates form. Lower limb buds are paddle-shaped.
16	9~10	5	Foot plates form. Pigment visible in retina.
17	11~14	5.5	Digital rays appear in the hand plates.
18	14~16	6	Digital rays appear in the foot plates. Finger rays are notched.
19	17~20	7	Limb extends forward. Straightening of the trunk.
20	21~23	7	Upper limbs become longer and bend at elbow. Notched between the digital rays in the foot.
21	22~24	7	Hands and feet approach each other. Fingers are free and longer.
22	25~27	8	Toes are free and longer.
23	28~30	9	Upper and lower limbs become longer.
	39~41	10	
	64~66	11	
	77~79	12	
	91~93	13	
	105~107	14	
	119~121	15	
	132~134	16	
	± 147	17	
	± 160	18	
	± 173	19	
	± 185	20	
	± 197	21	
	± 208	22	
	± 219	23	
	± 230	24	
	± 270	28	
	± 310	32	
	± 346	36	
	± 362	38	

* Streeter G. L. ; Developmental horizon in human embryos, Carnegie Institution of Washington, Washington D. C., 1959.

Contents

The Development of the Limb Buds

Chapter 01

The first mesenchymatous condensations of the appendicular skeleton are in the region of the future girdles and those for the pectoral region appear a little before those of the pelvic region. In their basic plan of structure, the arm and leg are closely comparable. The upper limb buds develop opposite the lower cervical segments, and the lower limb buds appear at the level of the lower lumbar segments. Each limb bud consists of an outer ectodermal cap and an inner mesodermal core. At the apex of each limb bud, the ectoderm thickens to form an apical ectodermal ridge (AER).

By the start of the fifth week, the upper limb buds are paddle-shaped and lower limb buds are flipper-like. At the start of the sixth week, the upper limbs begin to show regional differentiation as the elbows and hand plates (Figs. 1-1 and 1-2). The primordia of the fingers begin to develop in the hand plates, which indicate the formation of digits. At the tip of each digital ray, a part of the apical ectodermal ridge induces development of the mesenchyme into the mesenchymal primordia of the bones in the digits. The AER of the upper and lower limbs are first seen in the fifth week (Figs. 1-3 and 1-7) and disappear after the sixth week. Development of the lower limbs occurs somewhat later than that of the upper limbs (Fig. 1-7). During the fifth week, the peripheral nerves grow from the developing brachial and lumbosacral plexuses into the mesenchyme of the limb buds.

The mesenchyme in the limb bud gives rise to bones, ligaments, and blood vessels. By the start of the sixth week, the mesenchymal precursor of the distal limb skeleton is distinct in the upper and lower limbs, and chondrification commences in the humerus, ulna, and radius (Fig. 1-4). By the end of the sixth week, the carpal and metacarpal bones also begin to chondrify (Fig. 1-5). Nerves also advance and the radial, median, and ulna nerves reach the hand plate (Fig. 1-6). In the lower limb, the femur, tibia, and fibula begin to chondrify by the middle of the sixth week (Fig. 1-7), and tarsal and metatarsals begin to chondrify by the end of the sixth week (Fig. 1-8).

During the fifth week, the somitic mesoderm invades the limb bud and forms two large condensations, one ventral to the axial mesenchymal column and the other dorsal to it. The cell of the condensations forms the anlagen of the limb muscles and differentiates into myoblasts. As the long bones form, myoblasts fuse together to form a large muscle mass in each limb bud. In general, this muscle mass separates into dorsal and ventral components.

The primary ossification centers of the limb bones appear in the eighth week. By 12th week, primary ossification centers have appeared in nearly all bones in the limbs.

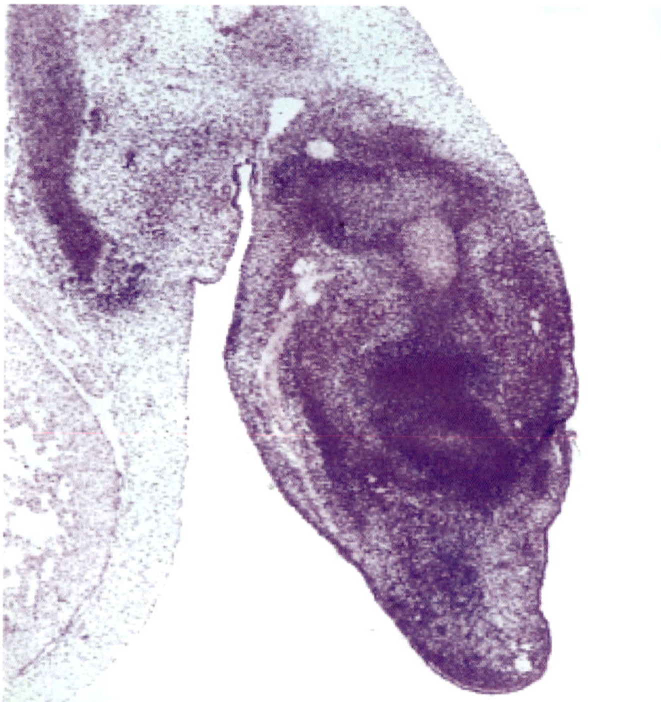

Fig. 1-1. Transverse section through the heart of a 11 mm CR length, Carnegie stage 17 embryo to show the development of the skeletal blastema. The cartilage models of humerus, ulna, and radius are seen. At the apex of the limb bud, the ectoderm thickens to form an apical ectoderm ridge (AER). Note the ulna nerve at the level of the elbow.

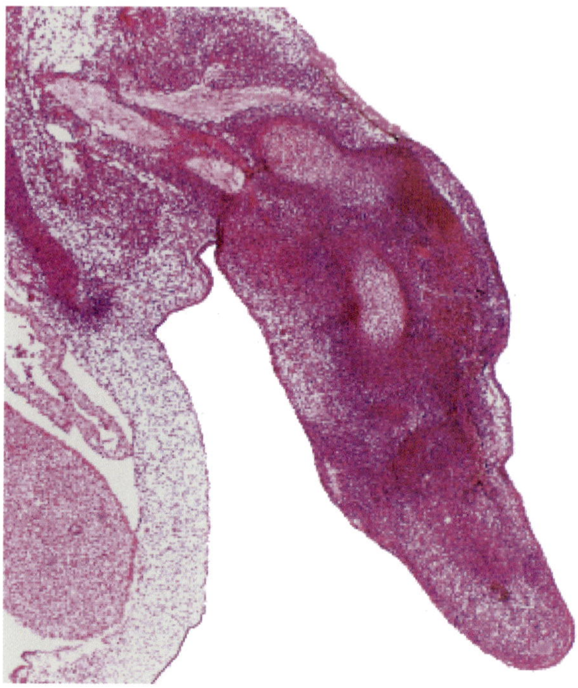

Fig. 1-2. Transverse section from a 11 mm embryo to show the skeletal blastema. The cartilage models of humerus and radius are clearly visible. Note the nerves entering the limb bud.

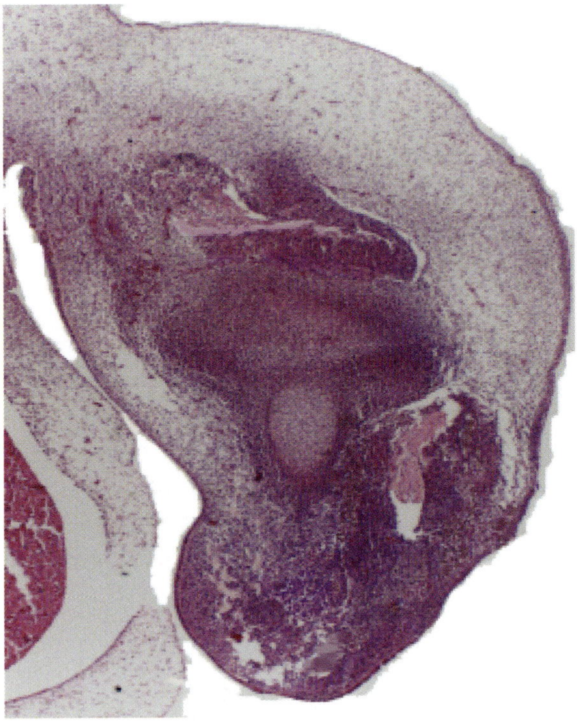

Fig. 1-3. Transverse section through the part of the liver level at 12 mm CR length, Carnegie stage 17 embryo to show the skeletal blastema of humeral and radial regions. At the tip of the limb bud the ectoderm thickens to form an apical ectodermal ridge. Nerves arising from the spinal cord grow into the muscle masses.

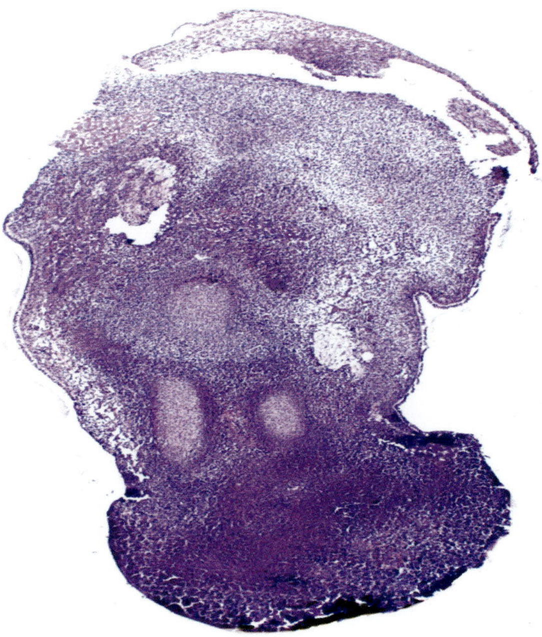

Fig. 1-4. Transverse section of the developing upper limb at 14 mm CR length, Carnegie stage 18 embryo to show the cartilaginous model of the humerus, radius, and ulna. Note the presence of two distinct nerves and apical ectodermal ridge.

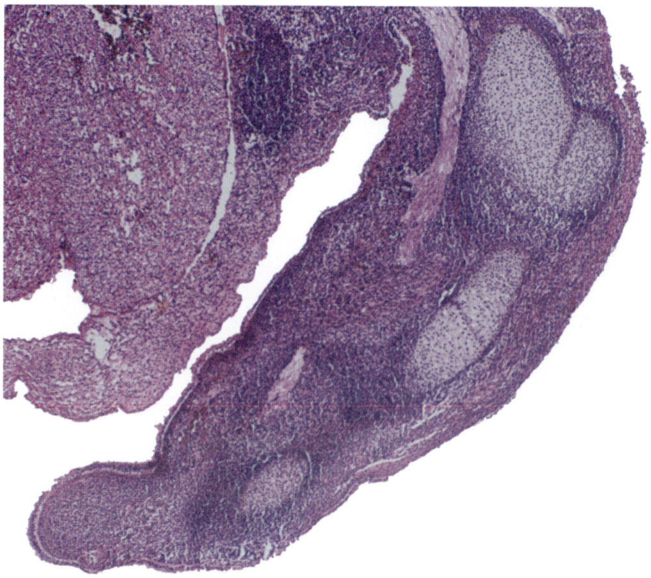

Fig. 1-5. Transverse section through the part of the liver level at 15 mm CR length, Carnegie stage 18 embryo to show development of the cartilaginous models of bones. Chondrification of the humerus and radius has started. The developing median nerve is visible.

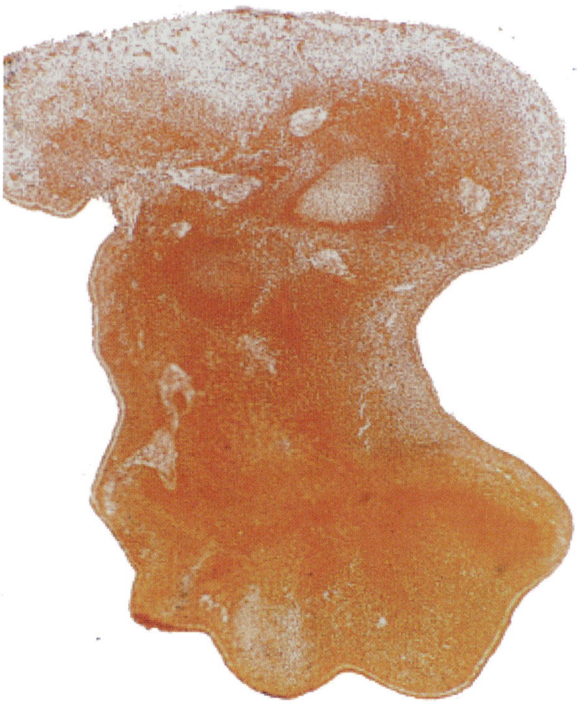

Fig. 1-6. Frontal section through the part of the upper limb bud at 16 mm CR length, Carnegie stage 19 embryo to show the outlines of the future digits.

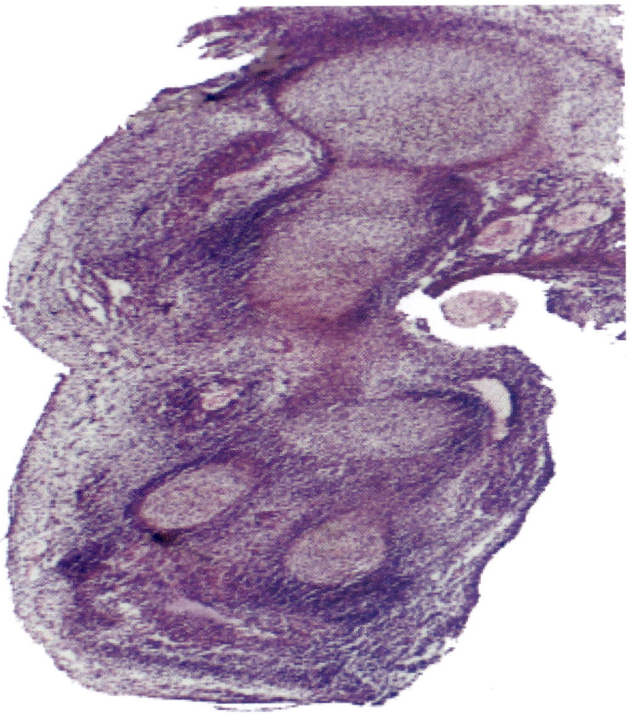

Fig. 1-7. Frontal section through the part of the lower limb bud at 17 mm CR length, Carnegie stage 19 embryo to show the skeletal blastema. The hip bone is chondrified and separated from the femur by a homogenous interzone. The tibia and fibula are well developed. The developing sciatic and femoral nerves are visible.

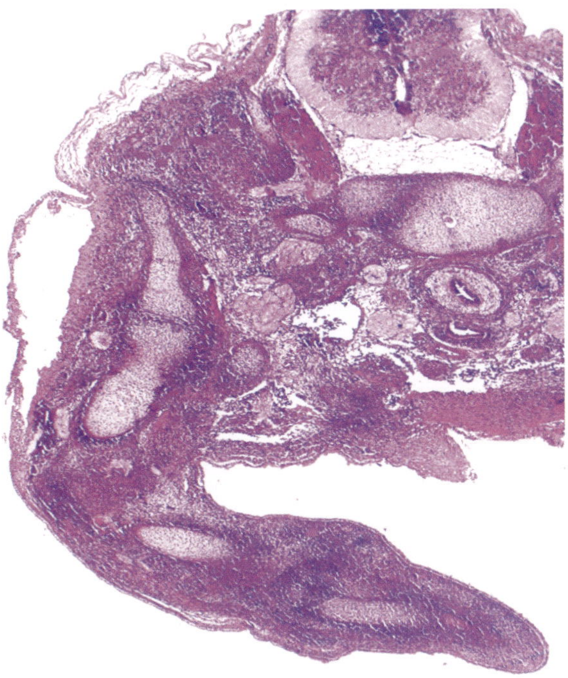

Fig. 1-8. Transverse section through the part of the ilium level at 18 mm CR length, Carnegie stage 20 embryo to show the cartilaginous models of the lower limb bud. Chondrifications of ilium, femur, tibia, and metatarsus are clearly visible. The cartilaginous anlage of a vertebra including the notochord is also seen.

References

O'Rahilly R, Gardner E: The timing and sequences of events in the development of the limbs in human embryo. *Anat Embryol* 148: 1-23, 1975.

Rutherford NC: A contribution to the embryology of the forelimb skeleton. *J Anat* 48: 355-377, 1914.

Streeter GI: Developmental horizons in the human embryos. A review of the histogenesis of cartilage and bone. *Contrib Embryol* 33: 151-168, 1949.

The Development of the Long Bones

Chapter 02

Most of the long bones of the body are developed by periosteal, endochondral and epiphyseal ossification.

Periosteal and endochondral ossification

The general shape of the femur is quite similar to that of the adult in a 20 mm embryo. Ossification begins at the middle of the cartilaginous model of the femur. A thin layer of the calcified bone matrix is laid down between the perichondrium and the portion of the shaft containing hypertrophied cartilage cells and by extending around the shaft forming a bony collar in the 25 mm embryo (Fig. 2-1), and in the 30 mm fetus it extends nearly one-fourth of the length of the femur (Fig. 2-2). This periosteal bone is in direct contact with cartilage. Simultaneously with the appearance of the bony collar, changes take place in the center of the diaphysis hypertrophy and become vacuolated. The hypertrophied chondrocytes result in the enlargement of their lacunae and reduction in the intervening cartilage matrix septa, which become calcified. Erosion of the bony collar is evident in the 40 mm fetus and destruction of the calcified cartilage occurs by the 45 mm fetus. Holes etched in the bony collar by osteoclasts permit a periosteal bud, composed of osteoprogenitor cells, and blood vessels, to enter the concavities within the cartilage model. These periosteal capillaries grow into the cartilage model and initiate the development of a primary center of ossification in the 50 mm fetus. This formation of bone constitutes endochondral ossification (Fig. 2-3). As endochondral ossification proceeds proximally and distally and growth zones become established, periosteal bone formation also proceeds longitudinally until the 260 mm fetus, and extends about 1-2 mm beyond the zone of cartilage destruction in the growth zones. After the 260 mm fetus, the extents of endochondral and periosteal ossification are the same and at term occupy 70% of the length of the femur. Trabeculation of the bony collar is first noted in the 50 mm fetus (Fig. 2-4). Fusion of endochondral trabeculae with the inner aspect of the periosteal shell begins by the 70 mm fetus (Figs. 2-5 and 2-6). Evidence of reconstruction appears in both the proximal and distal ends by the 105 mm fetus (Fig. 2-7) and is always present in both ends after the 120 mm fetus (Figs. 2-8. 2-9, and 2-10). The trabeculated compacta of the peristeal bone is thick and the marrow cavity is relatively narrow by the 150 mm fetus (Figs. 2-10 and 2-11).

Epiphseal ossification

Until skeletal growth is completed, a long bone continues to lengthen as a result of interstitial growth of the cartilage that is retained as its epiphyseal growth plates. Because the epiphyseal plates grow on one side and become replaced by bone on the other, they are gradually shifted apart, lengthening the bony diaphysis that lies between them (Fig. 2-12). The formation of long bones is slightly more complex because these bones develop the secondary center of ossification. The majority of secondary centers are formed postnatally, but those in the distal and proximal tibia begin to appear just prior to birth. The first morphological evidence of the developing secondary center of the ossification center in the distal femoral chondroepiphysis is found in the 300 mm fetus (Fig. 2-13). The ossification center is in the form of multiple foci of calcification. Initial calcification occurs immediately adjacent to the end of a cartilage canal and not an avascular matrix. Once the bony center appears, ossification along the articular side of the secondary center is different from that along the metaphyseal side. The hypertrophied chondrocytes of the articular side are not distinctly parallel and the intercellular matrix is mineralized in all directions. As the secondary center expands toward the metaphyseal side, many chondrocytes do not degenerate (Fig. 2-15). With the progressive development of the secondary ossification center, the epiphyseal growth plate becomes well differentiated and shows a typical zonal differentiation (Figs. 2-14 and 3-15). In the youngest child, the perichondral ring (membrane) extends well beyond the advancing trabeculae of the metaphysis and in the seven-year-old it extends only slightly beyond the adjacent trabeculae (Fig. 2-15). Throughout the period of active bone growth, the dense layer of the perichondral ring is demonstrated. These findings support the previous suggestion that the transverse diameter of the epiphyseal plate increases by appositional growth from the overlying perichondrium, and that the same source is responsible for the lateral extension of the articular cartilage during growth.

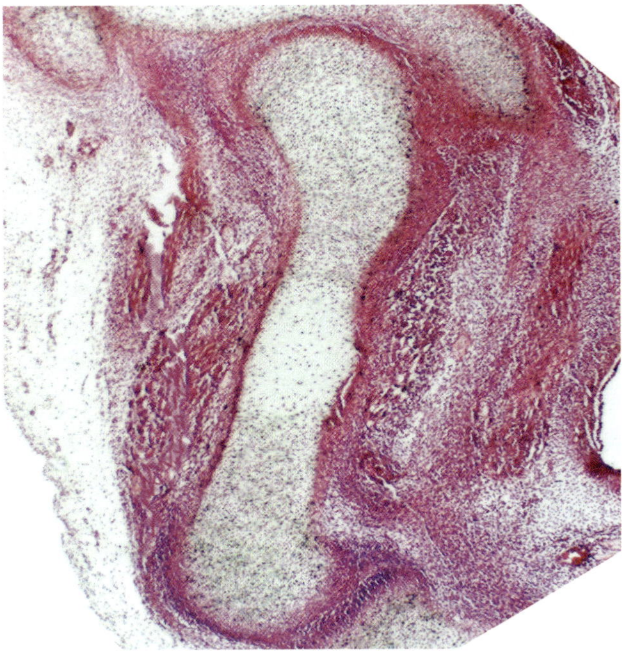

Fig. 2-1. Sagittal section of the femur from a 25 mm embryo to show the primary bony collar in the shaft. The hypertrophied chondrocytes in the center of the shaft prior to vascular irruption is seen.

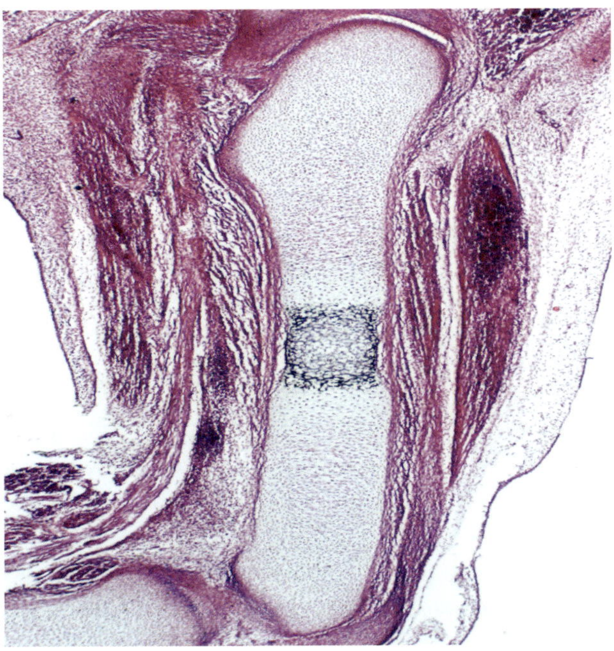

Fig. 2-2. Sagittal section of the femur from a 30 mm fetus to show the extent of ossification in the shaft. A bony collar extends for nearly one-fourth of the length of the femur.

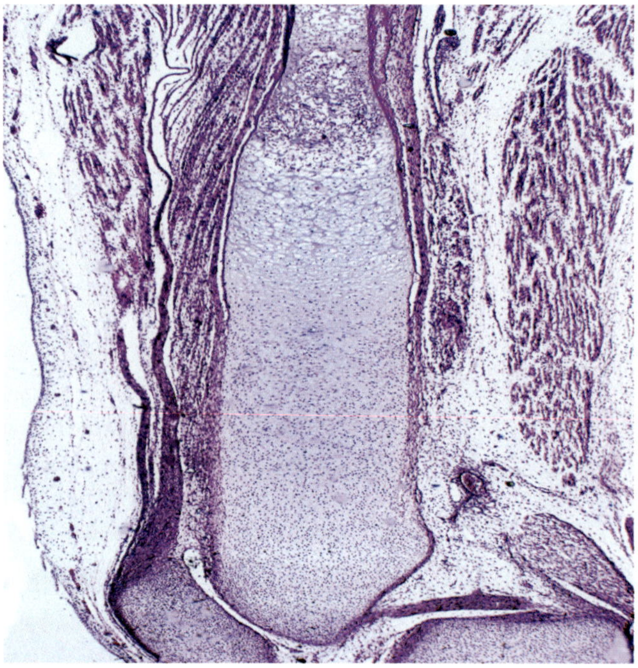

Fig. 2-3. Sagittal section through the part of the distal femur from a 50 mm fetus to show the extent of endochondral ossification. Periosteal bone extends proximally beyond the level of endochondral ossification.

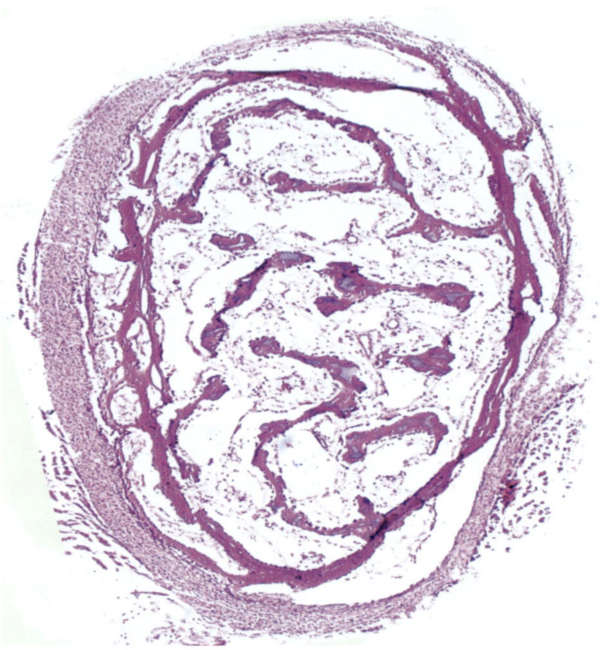

Fig. 2-4. Cross section through the shaft of the femur from a 50 mm fetus to show the endochondral trabeculae. Fusion of endochondral trabeculae with periosteally formed shell is seen.

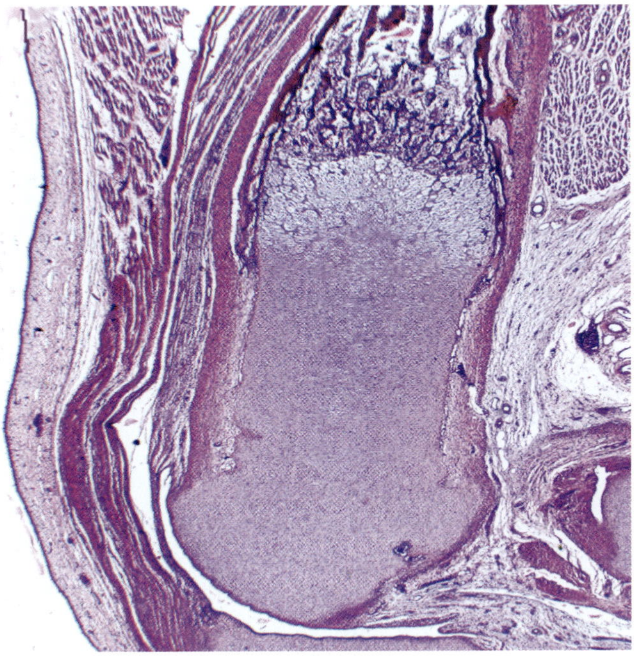

Fig. 2-5. Sagittal section of the distal femur from a 70 mm fetus to show zonal differentiation of the diaphyseal growing part of the cartilaginous epiphysis. Note the periosteal bone extending toward the lower end, ahead of endochondral ossification and at the same level as the zone of hypertrophied chondrocytes.

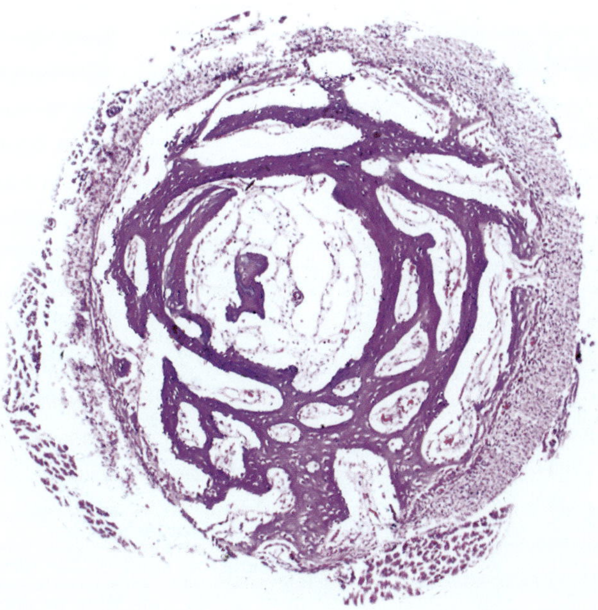

Fig. 2-6. Cross section through the shaft of the femur from a 70 mm fetus to show the linea aspera with marked periosteal bone formation.

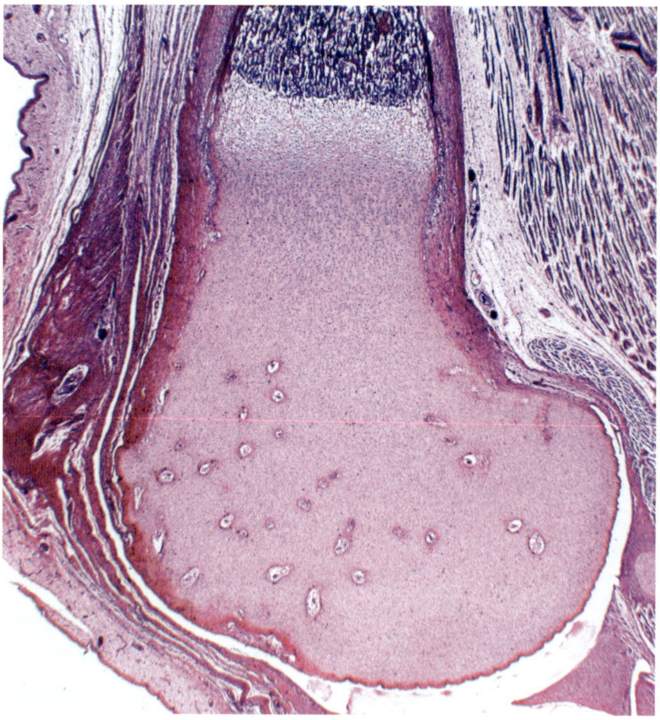

Fig. 2-7. Sagittal section of the lower femur from a 105 mm fetus to show many cartilage canals in the epiphysis.

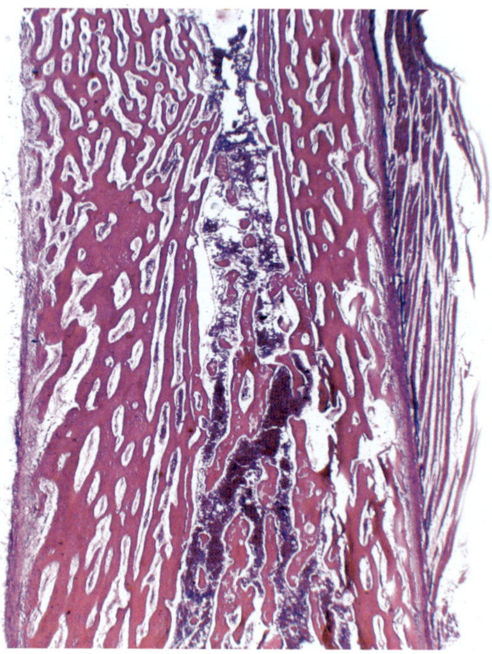

Fig. 2-8. Frontal section through the shaft of the femur from a 120 mm fetus to show the trabeculated periosteal compacta.

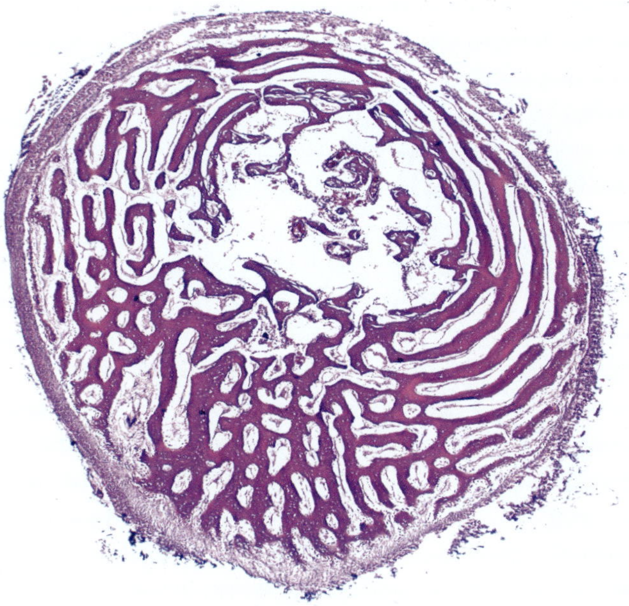

Fig. 2-9. Cross section through the shaft of the femur from a 120 mm fetus to show trabeculated compacta. Fusion of the endochondral trabeculae with the periosteal compacta is seen.

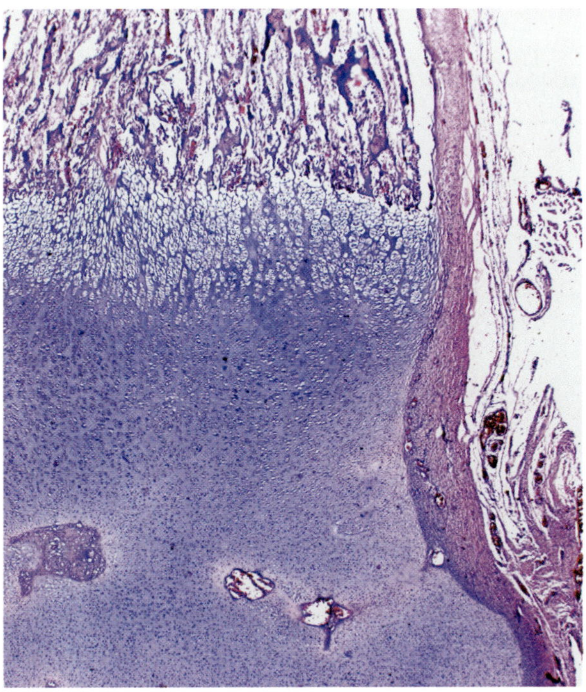

Fig. 2-10. Sagittal section through the part of the distal femur from a 150 mm fetus to show early a columnar arrangement of chondrocytes of the epiphyseal plate. The dense cell layer of the perichondral zone is separated from the epiphyseal plate.

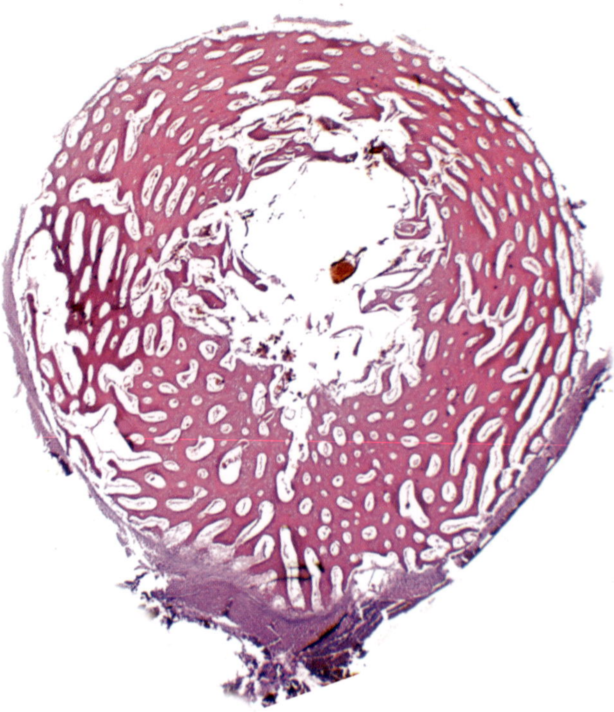

Fig. 2-11. Cross section through the part of the shaft of the femur from a 160 mm fetus to show trabeculated periosteal compacta and marrow cavity. Note the extensive removal of compacta lateral and medial to linea aspera.

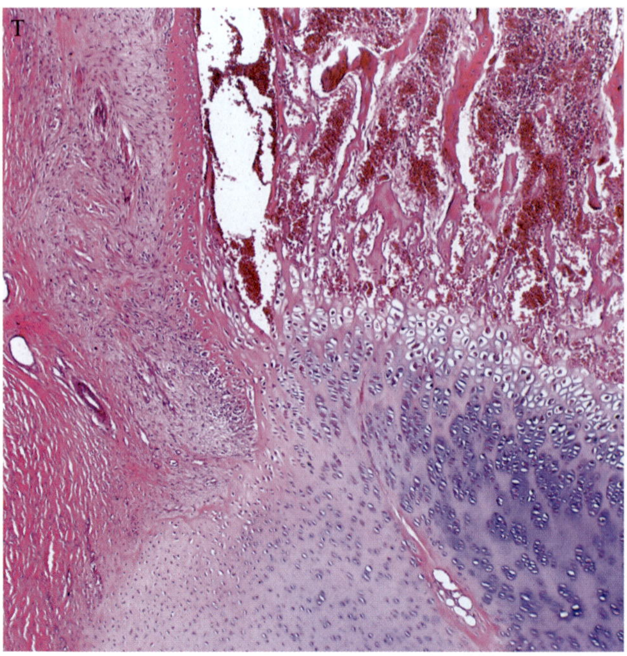

Fig. 2-12. Sagittal section through the part of the distal femur from a 200 mm fetus to show the perichondral zone. The marginal germinal zone is well seen. The perichondral ring (periosteal lamellae) is related to the hypertrophied chondrocytes of the growth plate. The dense cell layer of the perichondral zone is separated from the epiphyseal plate and from the marginal germinal zone.

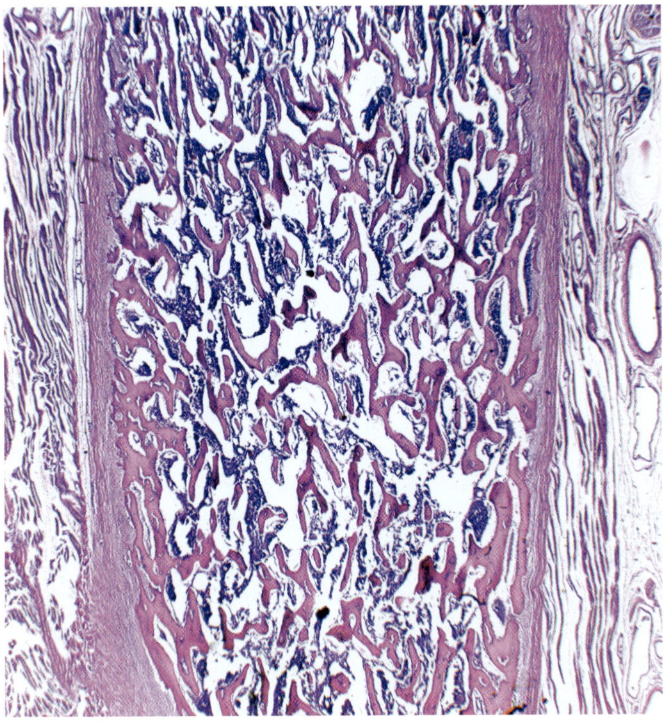

Fig. 2-13. Frontal section through the distal third of the femur from a 300 mm fetus to show endochondral trabeculae. Note the regular arrangement and layering of compacta.

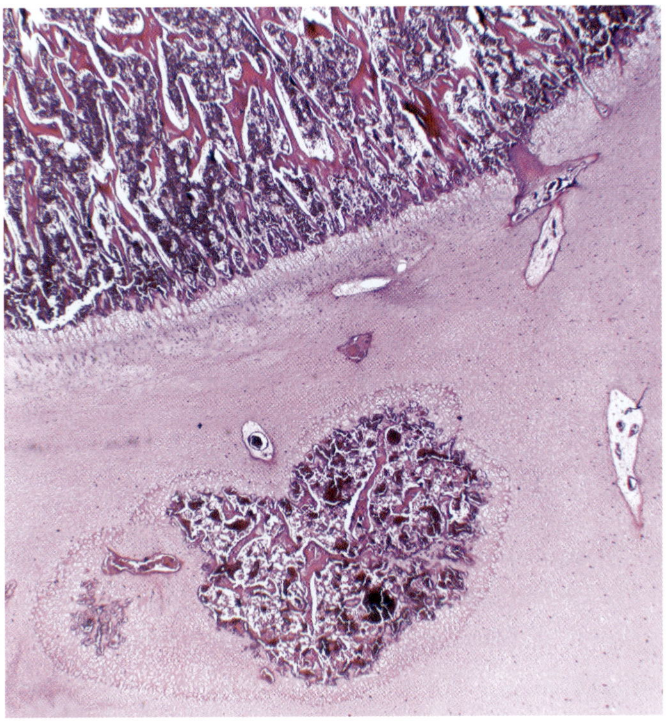

Fig. 2-14. Sagittal section through the part of the distal epiphysis of the femur in a 360 mm fetus to show the distinct zonal differentiation of the cartilaginous epiphysis. The layers of resting cartilage, proliferation, maturation, and calcification are noted. One cartilage canal crosses the physis. Note the development of the secondary center of ossification from the calcified foci to coalescence.

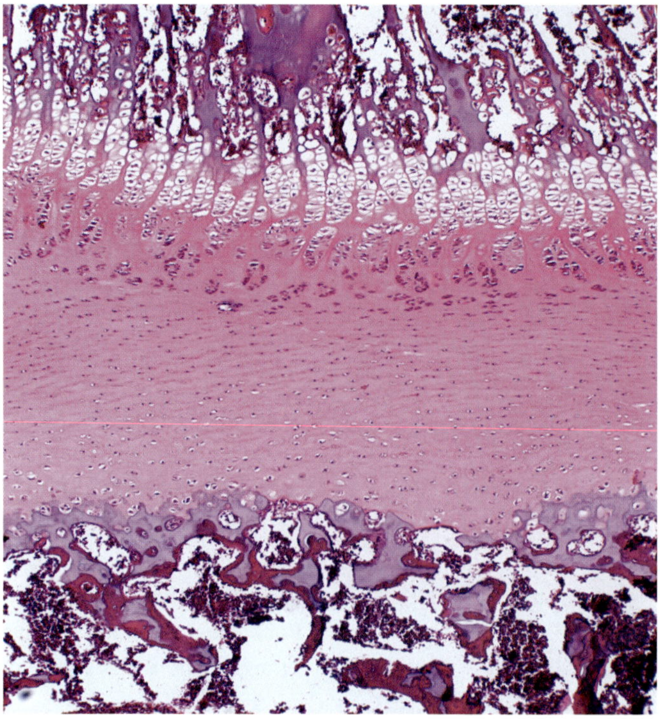

Fig. 2-15. Frontal section through the part of the distal epiphysis of the femur from 2 months after birth to show ossification along the metaphyseal side. Note many cartilage cells bordering the metaphyseal side of the bony center do not degenerate. The four layers of the epiphyseal plate are seen.

References

Bardeen C: Studies of the development of the human skeleton. *Am J Anat.* 4: 265-302, 1905.

Gardner E, O'Rahilly R: The early development of the knee joint in staged human embryos. *J Anat* 102: 289-299, 1968.

Gray DJ, Gardner E: Prenatal development of the human knee and superior tibiofibular joint. *Am J Anat* 86: 235-287, 1950.

Kuhlman RE: A microchemical study of the developing epiphyseal plate. *J Bone Joint Surg* 42A: 457-466, 1960.

Noback CR, Robertson GG: Sequences of appearance of ossification centers in the human skeleton during the first five prenatal months. *Am J Anat* 89: 1-28, 1951.

Park SL: The prenatal development of femur in Korean fetuses. *Chonnam Medical J* 10: 1075-1090, 1973.

Pratt CWM: Observations on osteogenesis in the femur of the foetal rat. *J Anat* 91: 533-544, 1957.

The Development of the Joint

Chapter 03

The differentiation of the joint is related to that of the bone segments which appear in the limb buds sucessively in a proximodistal direction. In the 12 mm embryo, the cartilages at the hand begin to adopt their characteristic shapes and the primitive joint plates (articular disk) are quite distinct, each formed by a mass of undifferentiated blastemal tissue between the cartilages (Fig. 3-1). Between the apposed ends of such developing cartilage models, the mesenchyme condenses and forms a homogenous interzone in the 20 mm embryo (Fig. 3-2). During the next phase, the three-layered interzone can be distinguished. This phenomenon is seen in all joints, the separation into three layers appearing first in large and proximal joints of the extremities. So far, there seems to be agreement between the various groups of investigators. The disagreement concerns the formation and time of formation of the joint cavities. The homogenous interzone in the joint is composed of a single cell type characterized by a large nucleus and a sparse cytoplasm. The interzone is differentiated into a three-layered interzone with two chondrogenous layers and an intermediate layer. In the early developmental stage, the intermediate layer of interzone consists of a zone which is 3-4 elongate cells thick, but in a later phase the cells are converted into chondroblast and incorporated into the chondrogenous layer. The cells of the intermediate layer of the interzone are arranged with their long axes at right angles to the long axes of the adjoining cartilages, and here mitotic figures are not as abundant as in the two chondrogenous layers. Three-layered interzones in the metacarpophalangeal joint is found in the 35 mm fetus (Fig. 3-3). This interzone is three-layered, consisting of two chondrogenous layers each continuing in the perichondrium of the cartilage, and in an intermediate layer of loose avascular mesenchyme which continues peripherally in a vascular mesenchyme (Fig. 3-4). In the 40 mm fetus, the primitive joint spaces are first seen in the three-layered interzone as a narrow cleft around the periphery (Fig. 3-5) and is completed between the 50 and 60 mm fetuses (Figs. 3-6 and 3-7). No degenerative phenomena of the intermediate layer of interzone are noticed. This investigation reveals that the formation of the joint cavity at the periphery in the joints after the intermediate layer of the interzone has become incorporated into the two chondrogenous layers of the interzone. By the 60-100 mm fetuses, most of the joints have attained the proportions they will have in the adult, and the synovial surfaces are formed of one or two layers of typical synovial cells lying on the vascular substratum (Figs. 3-8 and 3-9). With the further spread of the synovial cavities, a large proportion of the perichondrium becomes chondrified so as to form articular cartilages (Fig. 3-10). Near the margins of the articular surfaces, there is a marginal transitional zone between the articular surfaces and the perichondrium (Figs. 3-11 and 3-12).

With further development, the superficial chondrocytes are flattened, whereas both intermediate and deep chondrocytes are ovoid or spherical (Fig. 3-13). After the 200 mm fetus, the synovial membrane may classify the synovium as fatty, areolar, and fibrous types based upon the nature of the subintimal tissues (Fig. 3-14).

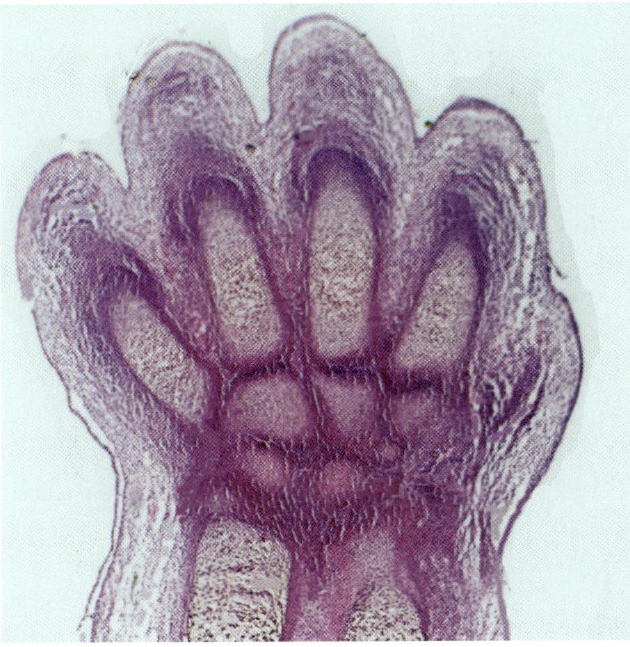

Fig. 3-1. Frontal section through the part of the hand in a 12 mm embryo, Carnegie stage 17, showing the primitive joint plate. The carpal and carpometacarpal regions are represented by masses of condensed blastema.

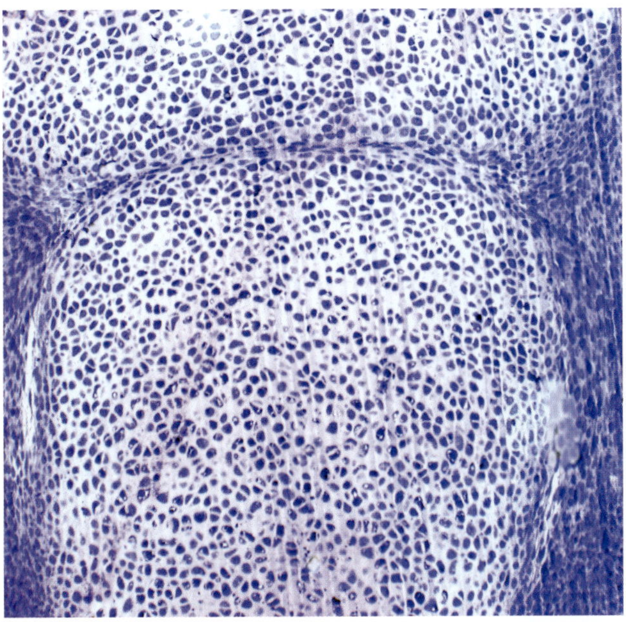

Fig. 3-2. Frontal section through the part of the metacarpophalangeal joint from a 20 mm embryo, Carnegie stage 20, showing the homogenous interzone. The condyles of the proximal phalanx are separated from the metacarpal bone by homogenous interzone.

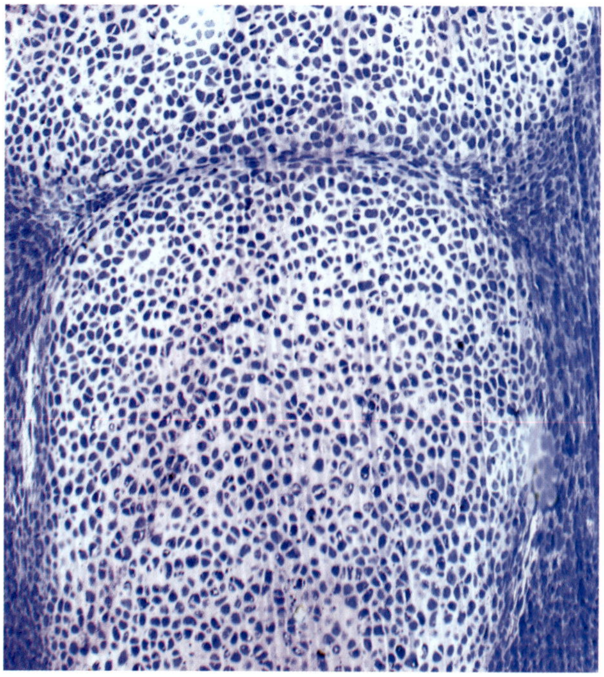

Fig. 3-3. Frontal section through the part of the metacarpophalangeal joint in the 35 mm fetus to show the three-layered interzone. The three-layered interzone with its chondrogenous layers and intermediate is shown fully developed between the phalanx and metacarpal bone. The chondrogenous layers are continued into the perichondrium, and the intermediate layer into the synovial mesenchyme.

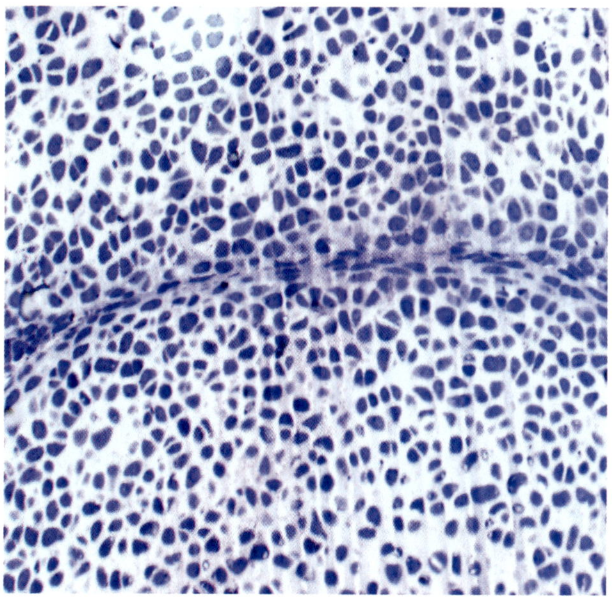

Fig. 3-4. High magnification of Fig. 4-3, showing a discontinuous line of elongated cells in the intermediate layer which traces a path of joint clefting.

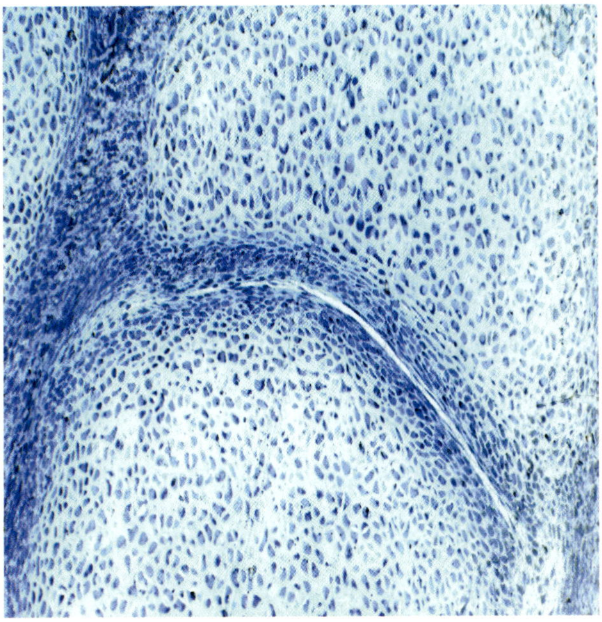

Fig. 3-5. Frontal section through the part of the metacarpophalangeal joints from a 40 mm fetus to show peripheral cavitation of the joint. The articular surface is smooth, and the chondrogenous layers are thick.

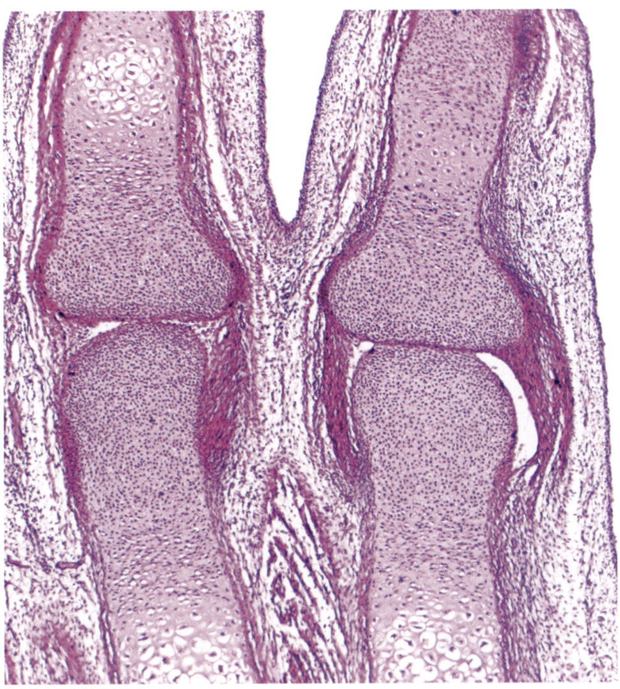

Fig. 3-6. Frontal section through the part of the hand in the 50 mm fetus to show complete formation of the metacarpophalangeal joints. The joint cavity appears partially obliterated, probably as a result of compressing during preparation. Note the collateral ligaments.

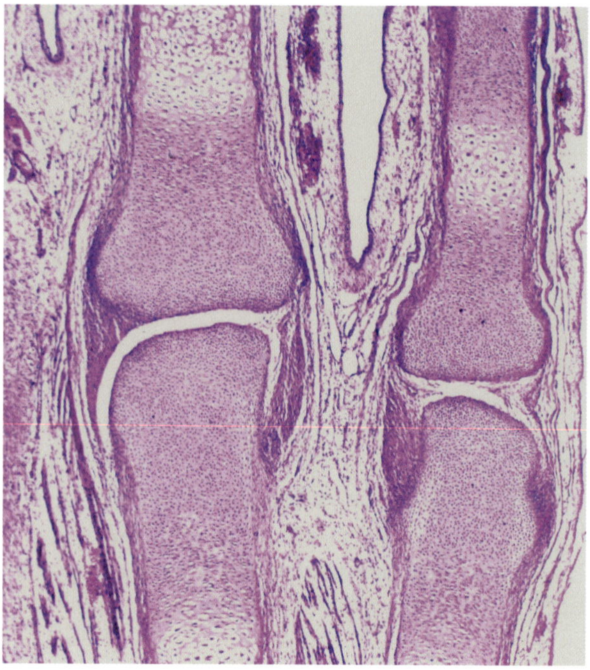

Fig. 3-7. Frontal section through the part of the hand from a 60 mm fetus to show the well developed cavity of metacarpophalangeal joints. A portion of the synovial fold projects into the joint cavity.

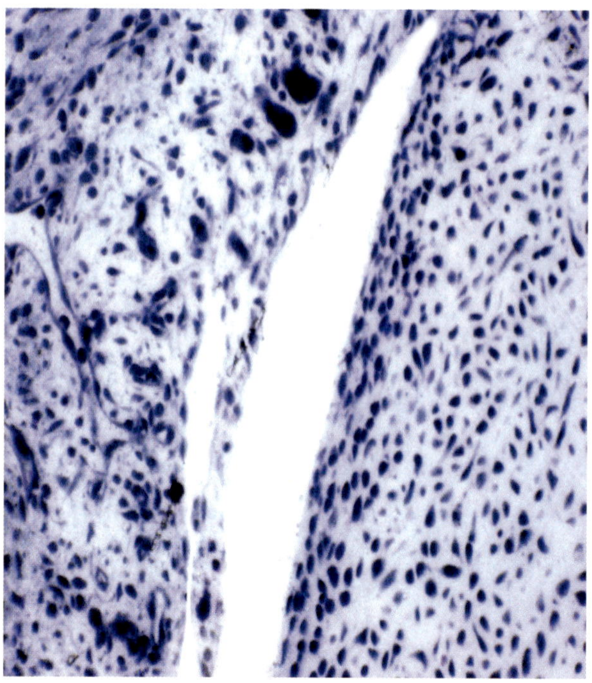

Fig. 3-8. Frontal section through the part of the hand from a 60 mm fetus to show the synovial membrane and articular cartilage. The articular surfaces are smooth. Superficial cells are large and discoidal, while deep cells are ovoid. Note early villus projects into cavity from an angle of synovial reflection.

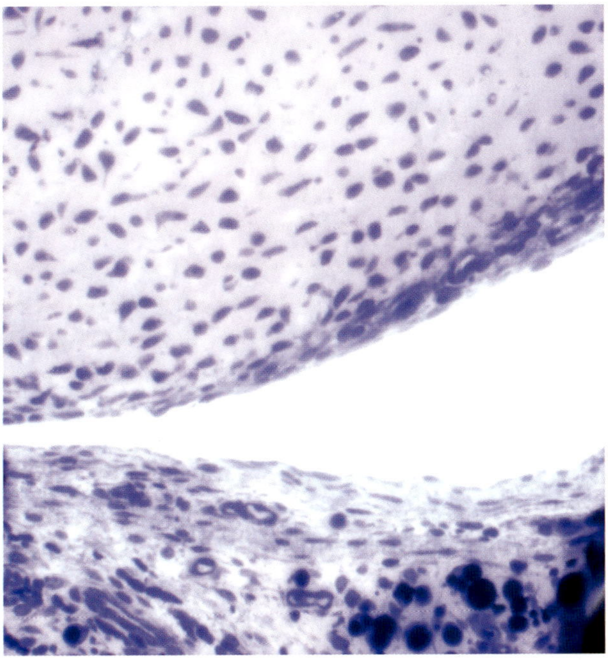

Fig. 3-9. Frontal section through the part of the metacarpophalangeal joint in the 100 mm fetus to show the synovial membrane. Synovial intimal cells are formed by a single row of cells. Synovial intima and subintima show well-organized collagen fiber in the subintima and capillaries abutting the synovial intima.

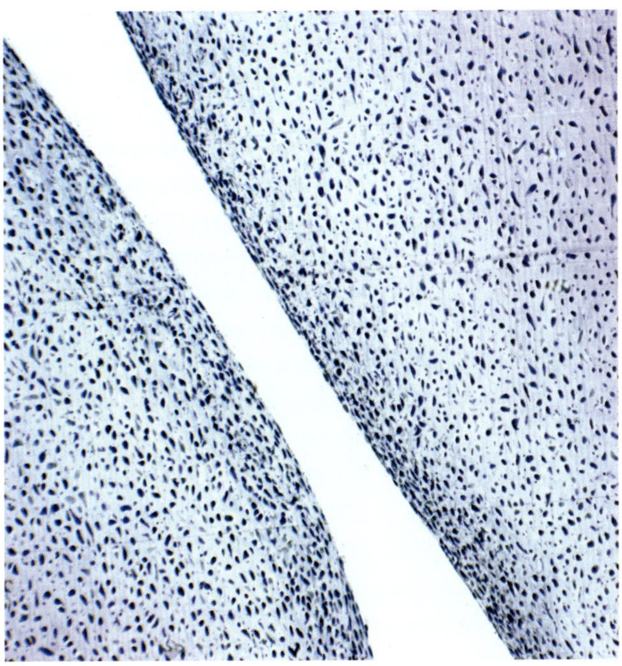

Fig. 3-10. Frontal section through the part of the metacarpophalangeal joint from a 120 mm fetus to show the articular cartilage. Superficial cells are small and flattened. In both the intermediate and deep zones, the cells are still round.

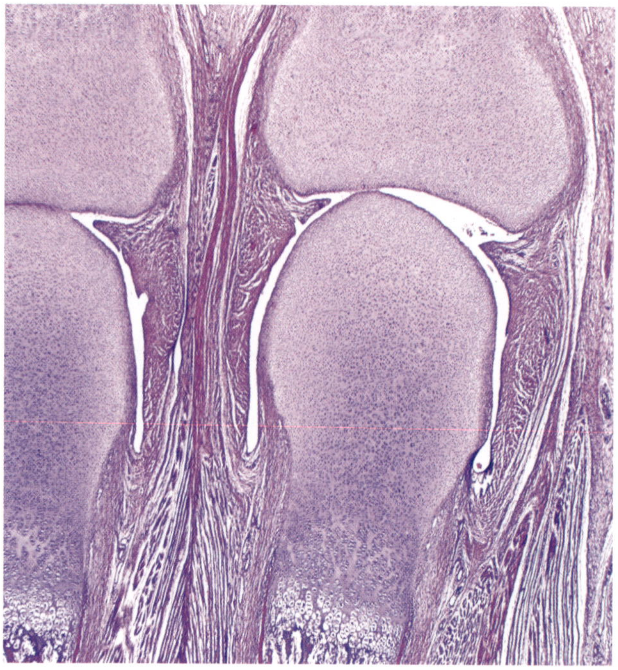

Fig. 3-11. Frontal section through the part of the hand in a 100 mm fetus to show vascular synovial fold in the metacarpophalangeal joint.

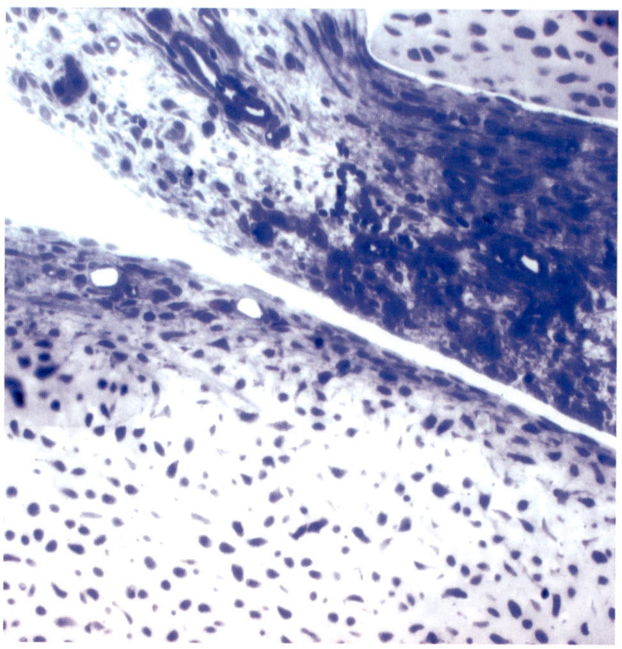

Fig. 3-12. Frontal section through the part of the metacarpophalangeal joint from a 160 mm fetus to show the articular cartilage and synovial membrane. Synovial intimal cells are widely separated from one another and look like the underlying fibroblasts. The superficial zone of articular cartilage contains small and flattened chondrocytes. In the deep part, the chondrocytes are ovoid or spherical. Note the marginal transitional zone between the articular cartilage and perichondrial tissues.

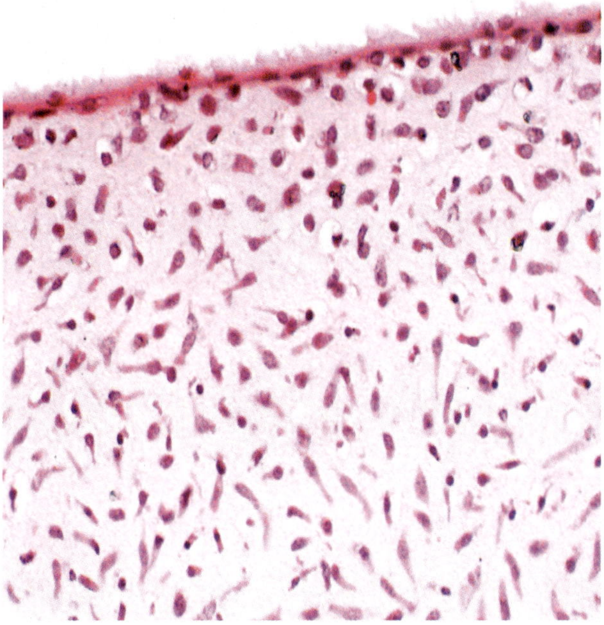

Fig. 3-13. Frontal section through the part of the metacarpophalangeal joint from a 200 mm fetus to show articular chondrocytes. In the superficial zone, the chondrocytes are flattened. In both intermediate and deep zones, the cells are arranged in columns lying oblique and perpendicular to the surface.

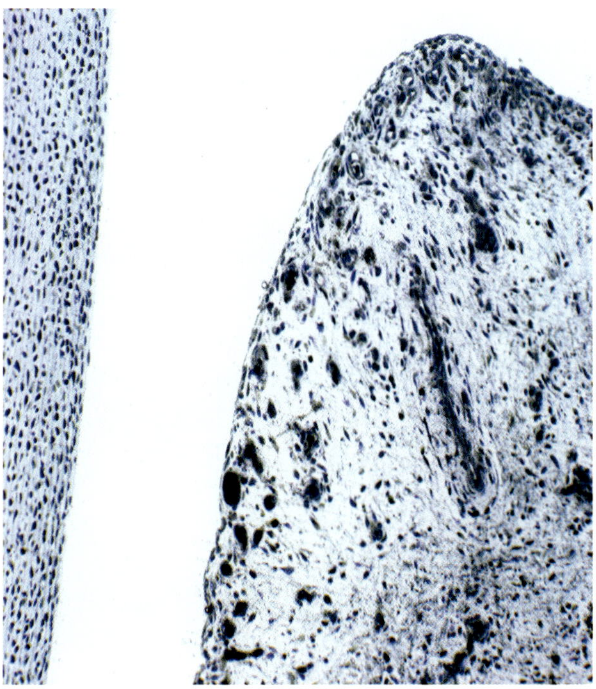

Fig. 3-14. Frontal section through the part of the hand region from a 200 mm fetus to show the articular cartilage and synovial membrane. Adjacent to the joint space lies the synovial intima which is three or four cells deep. The loose connective tissue comprising the subintima contains several blood vessls.

References

Andersen H, Bro-Rasmussen F: Histochemical studies on the histogenesis of the joints in human foetuses with special reference to the development of joint cavity in the hand and foot. *Am J Anat* 108: 111-122, 1961.

Bardeen CR: Studies of the development of the human skeleton. *Am J Anat* 4: 265-302, 1905.

Gardner E, Gray DJ, O'Rahilly R: The prenatal development of the skeleton and joint of the human foot. *J Bone Joint Surg* 41A: 847-879, 1956.

Haines RW: The development of joint. *J Anat (London)* 81: 33-55, 1947.

Mitrovic D: Development of the metatarsophalangeal joint of the chick embryo: morphological, ultrastructural, and histochemical studies. *Am J Anat* 150: 333-348, 1977.

Mitrovic D: Development of the diarthrodial joints in the rat embryo. *Am J Anat* 151: 475-486, 1978.

Moon EJ: Ultrastructure on histogenesis of the synovial joints in human fetuses. *Chonnam Medical J* 22: 451-463, 1985.

O'Rahilly R: The development of the synovial joint in the chick. *Anat Rec* 112: 303-375, 1952.

The Early Development of the Vertebrae

Chapter 04

During early embryonic period, somites soon diferentiate into a ventrolateral part, the sclerotome, and a dorsolateral part, the dermatomyotome. In the 4th week of development, the cells of sclerotomes shift their position to surround both the spinal cord and notochord. Each sclerotome consists of loosely arranged cells cranially and densely-packed cells caudally. Between sclerotomes, an intervertebral artery is present. Some densely-packed cells move cranially opposite the center of myotome, where they form the intervertebral disc. The remaining densely-packed cells fuse with the loosely-arranged cells of the immediately caudal sclerotome to form the future vertebral body or centrum. The primordia of the vertebrae in the 7 mm embryo are blastemal, and the primordia of the intervertebral disc can be distinguished from those of the body of the vertebrae by the cell populations in unit area, which are greater in the former than the latter (Fig. 4-1). The mesenchymal cells, surrounding the neural tube, form the vertebral (neural) arch in the 11 mm embryo (Fig. 4-3).

In a 8 mm embryo, the primordia of the vertebrae develop from the caudal sclerotome half of one segment and the cranial sclerotome half of the next succeeding segment (Fig. 4-2). Mesenchymal tissues, derived from the denser portion of the vertebral primordium, condense into an intervertebral disc within each interspace (Fig. 4-5), and the intersegmental arteries lie on each side of the vertebral bodies (Fig. 4-4). A pair of chondrification centers develops in each centrum (Figs. 4-6 and 4-7) and very soon these fuse across the midline to form the cartilaginous vertebral body by the 16 mm embryo (Figs. 4-8 and 4-9). The anulus fibrosus is noted as densely aggregated cells about each pole of the sclerotome in a 20 mm embryo (Fig. 4-10). Chondrification of the mesenchymal vertebra is completed by the 22 mm embryo (Fig. 4-11). By the time chondrification is completed, the rib cartilage becomes separated from the vertebra by the development of the primitive costocentral interzone (Fig. 4-12). During the mesenchymal or precartilaginous stage, the notochord degenerates and disappears, where it is surrounded by the developing vertebral bodies. Between the vertebrae, the notochord expands to form the gelatinous center of the intervertebral disc and the nucleus pulposus.

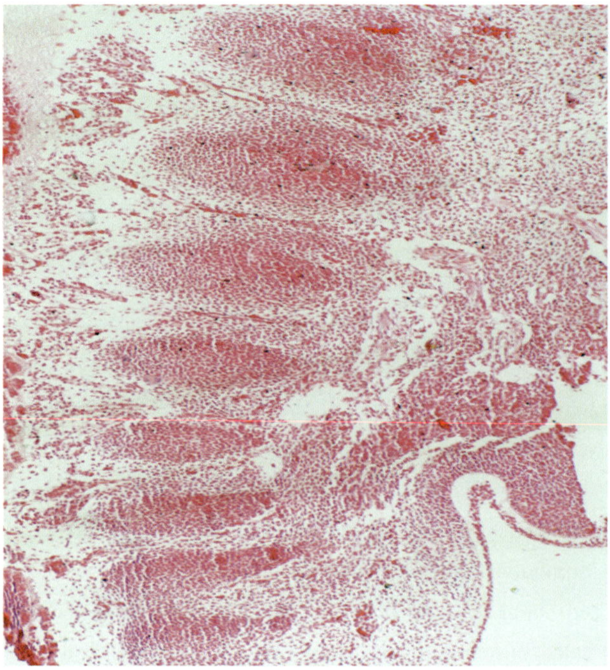

Fig. 4-1. Sagittal section, 7 mm, stage 15 embryo, showing the condensation of sclerotomal cells around the notochord consisted of a cranial area of loosely arranged cells and a caudal area of densely packed cells. Note the intersegmental artery in the area of the loosely arranged cells.

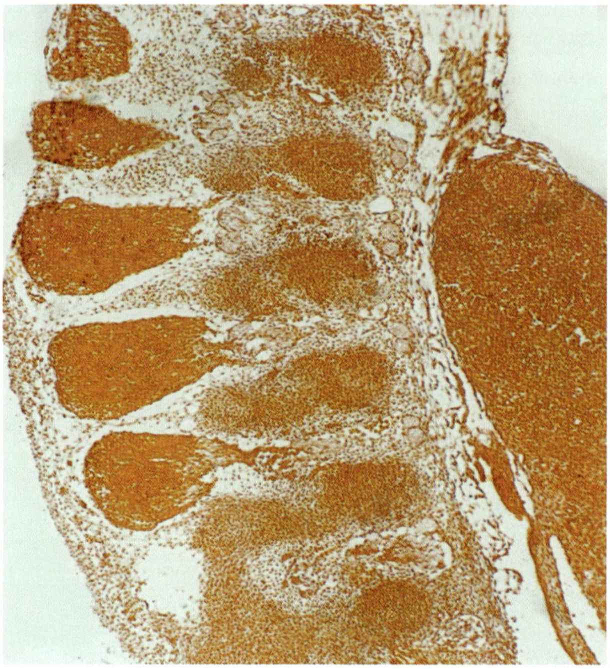

Fig. 4-2. Sagittal section through the level of the spinal ganglia of a 8 mm embryo, showing the developing vertebral column. The spinal ganglia lie behind the loosely-arranged cranial portion of the sclerotomes. Cranial to the loosely-arranged cranial portion, the intersegmental artery can be seen.

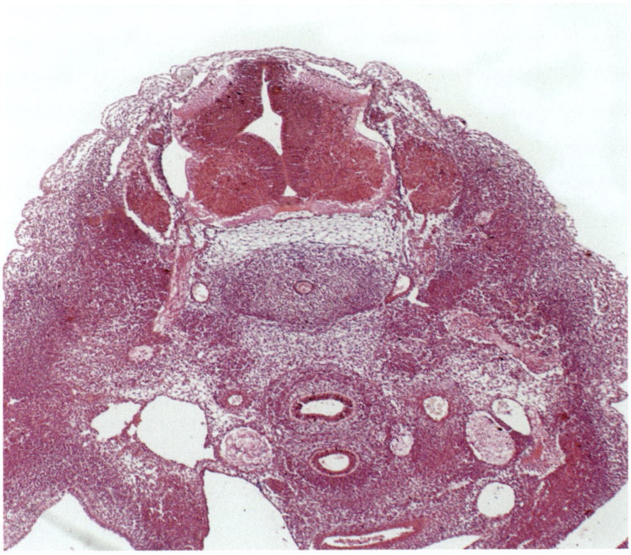

Fig. 4-3. Transverse section, 11 mm, stage 17 embryo, showing the condensation of sclerotomal cells around the notochord and neural tube.

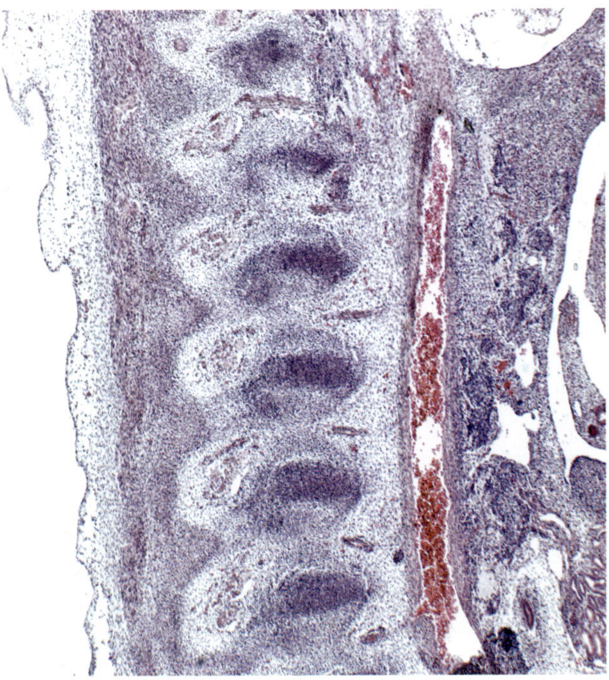

Fig. 4-4. Sagittal section, 11 mm, stage 17 embryo, showing a developing vertebral column. The intervertebral artery lies between the dense-celled area cranially and the loose-celled area caudally. The aorta is on the right.

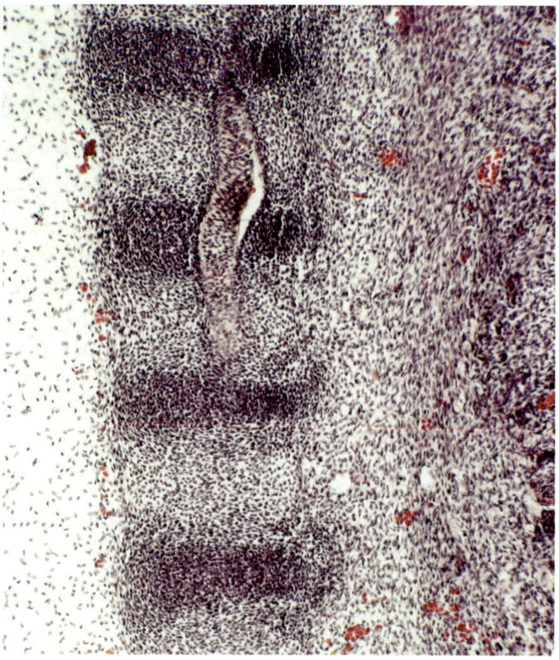

Fig. 4-5. Sagittal section through the midline of the vertebral body in a 14 mm, stage 18 embryo, showing definitive vertebrae. The denser area constitutes primodia of the intervertebral disc. The notochord and vertebral bodies are clearly shown.

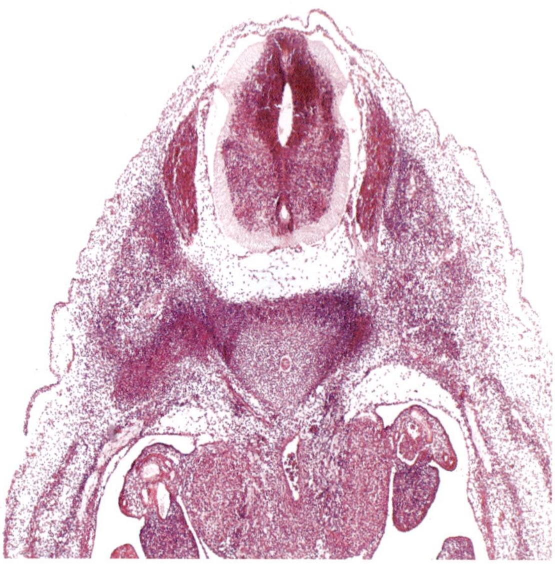

Fig. 4-6. Transverse section through the spinal cord region in a 14 mm, stage 18 embryo to show early chondrification in a mesenchymal vertebrae. Dorsal root ganglia and spinal cord are shown.

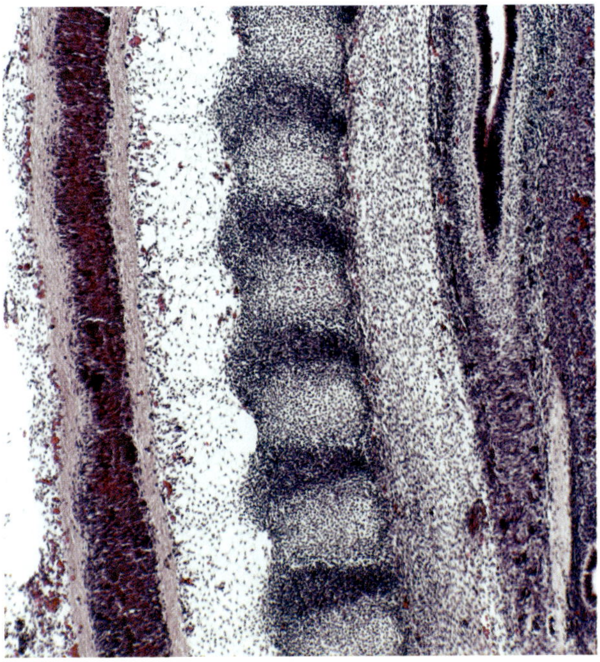

Fig. 4-7. Sagittal section through the midline of the cervical portion in a 14 mm, stage 18 embryo, showing the neural tube and definitive vertebrae. Note the oblique position of the vertebral bodies and intervertebral discs.

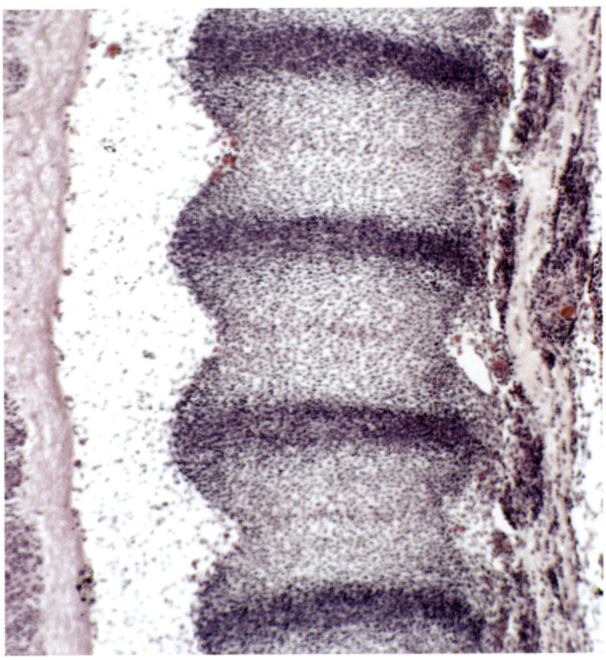

Fig. 4-8. Sagittal section through the midline of the thoracic portion from a 16 mm, stage 19 embryo, showing the definitive vertebrae. The densely-packed mesenchymal cells constitute the intervertebral discs.

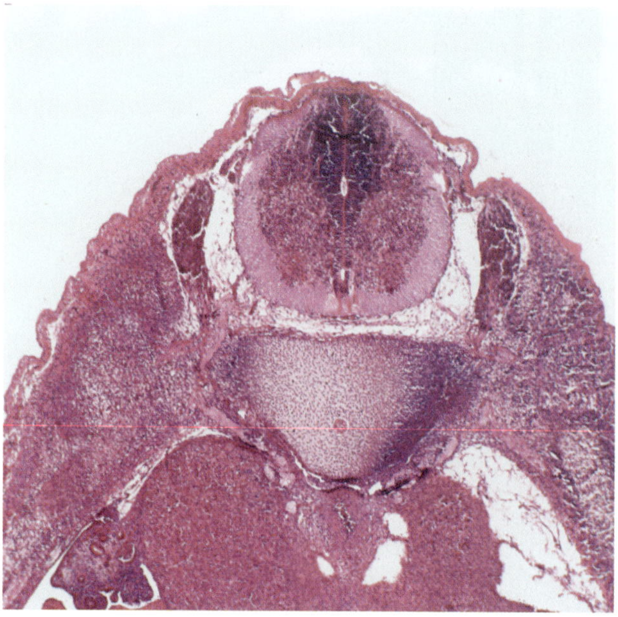

Fig. 4-9. Transverse section through the spinal cord region of a 16 mm, stage 19 embryo, showing chondrification of the vertebral body. The spinal cord and two dorsal spinal ganglia are shown.

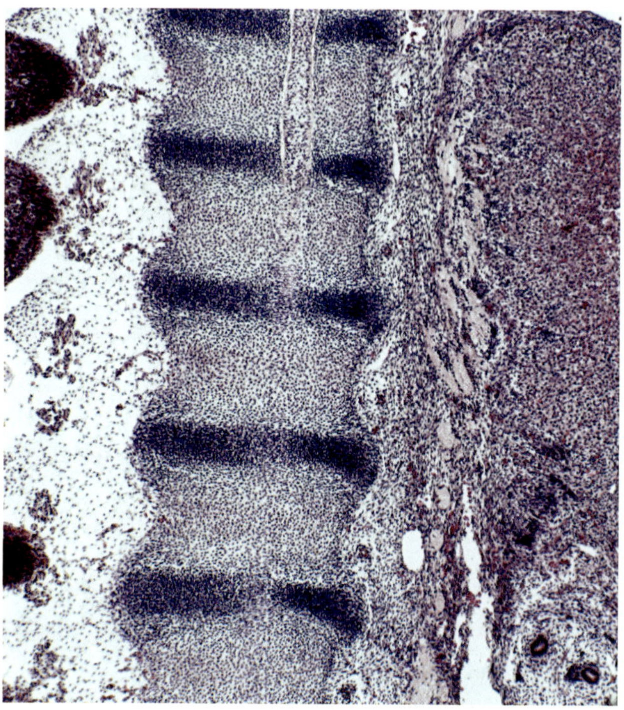

Fig. 4-10. Sagittal section through the midline of the vertebral body of a 20 mm, stage 20 embryo, showing the notochord and definitive vertebrae. The notochord is degenerating except in the region of the intervertebral disc, where it forms the nucleus pulposus. Note at the periphery the beginning of the formation of the anulus fibrosus.

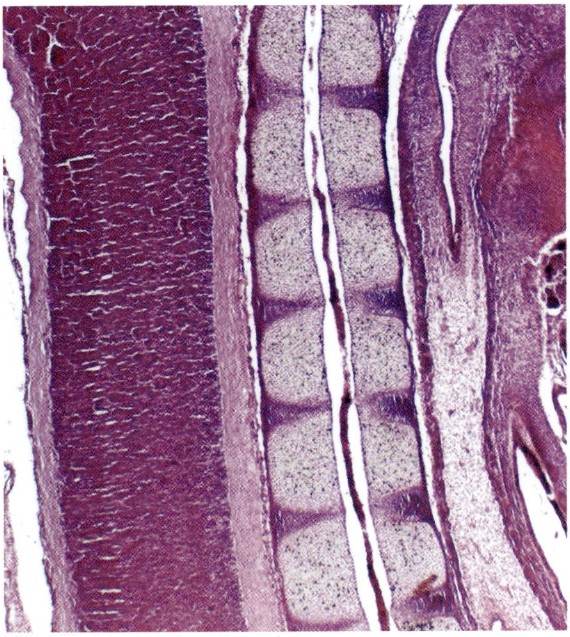

Fig. 4-11. Sagittal section through the midline of the vertebral body in a 22 mm, stage 21 embryo, showing vertebral bodies, neural tube, and notochord.

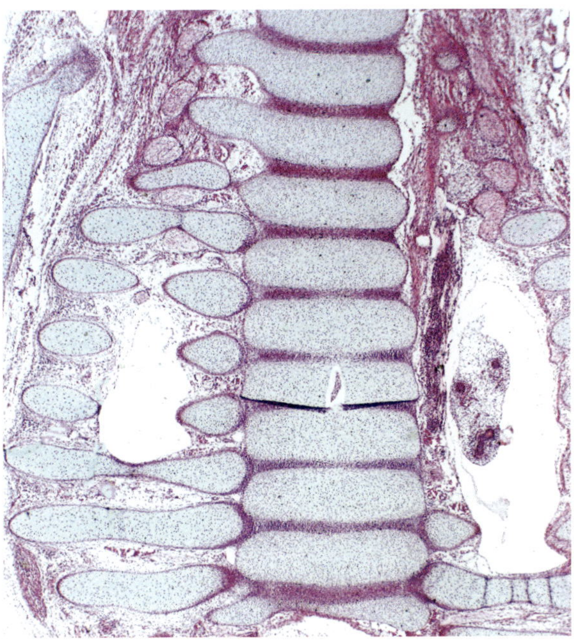

Fig. 4-12. Transverse section through the spinal cord in the upper thoracic region of a 23 mm, stage 22 embryo, showing chondrification of the vertebral bodies and ribs. The interzone between the vertebral body and the head of the rib is in the early homogenous stage.

References

Bick EM, Copel JN: Longitudinal growth of human vertebra. *J Bone Joint Surg* 32A: 803-814, 1950.

Han DY: The prenatal development of the vertebral column in Korean fetuses. *Chonnam Medical J* 6: 61-75, 1969.

O'Rahilly R, Meter DB: The timing and sequence of events in the development of the human vertebral column during the embryonic period proper. *Anat Embryol* 157: 167-179, 1979.

Peacock A: Observation on the prenatal development on the intervertebral disc in man. *J Anat* 85: 260-274, 1951.

Sensenig EC: The early development of the human vertebral column. *Contrib Embryol Carnegie Inst* 33: 21-41, 1949.

The Development of the Cervical Vertebrae

Chapter 05

In the 7 mm embryo, the sclerotomes appear as paired condensations of mesenchymal cells around the notochord and neural tube. Each sclerotome consists of loosely arranged cells cranially and densely arranged cells caudally. Mesenchymal tissues, derived from the densely arranged cells, condense into an intervertebral disc within each interspaces (Fig. 4-1). The intervertebral discs are distributed with six discs in the cervical region. The discs are structurally characterized by three integrated tissues: the nucleus pulposus, the anulus fibrosus, and cartilage end plates.

In the 14 mm embryo, chondrification centers appear in each mesenchymal vertebra. The two centers in each centrum fuse at the end of the embryonic period to form a cartilaginous centrum (Fig. 5-1). By the 24 mm embryo, the general form of the cervical vertebrae resembles that of the adult (Figs. 5-4 and 5-6). The cartilage canals of the cervical vertebrae are first seen in the 60 mm fetus (Fig. 5-8). Cartilage canals are identified as vascular channels arising from perichondrium surfaces. A number of cartilage canals are observed around the primary center of ossification in the 90 mm fetus (Fig. 5-10). By the 120 mm fetus, cartilage canals of the bodies of vertebra are increased (Fig. 5-11). Superficial, intermediate, and deep canals are identified by the characteristics of the cartilage cells and matrix surrounding the canals (Fig. 5-12). The vascular osteogenic tissue to the developing ossification center of the vertebra is provided by the adjoining cartilage canals.

With the exception of the first, second, and seventh vertebrae, the ossification centers of the cervical vertebrae, one in each arch and one in the body, are observed in the 80 mm fetus. The vertebral body starts to ossify two weeks later. The processes of bone formation in the vertebral bodies are found to process morphological similarities to that occurring at the secondary center of the epiphysis of a long bone (Fig. 5-12).

Atlanto-Axial Joint

In the 7 mm embryo, primordium of the atlas develops from the lower half of the first cervical sclerotome and the upper half of the second cervical sclerotome. The body of the axis is formed by the lower half of the second cervical sclerotome and upper half of the third cervical sclerotome. Fusion of the cartilaginous atlas and axis is observed in the 24 mm embryo (Fig. 5-5). By the 30 mm fetus, the general shape of the skeletal elements of the dens resembles that of the adult (Fig. 5-7). In the axis, chondrification begins in the body and arch in the 15 mm embryo (Fig. 5-2), and in the dens in the 24 mm embryo (Fig. 5-3).

Homogenous and three-layered interzones in the median atlantoaxial joint are observed in the 24 mm and 30 mm embryos, respectively (Figs. 5-5 and 5-7). Primitive joint cavities of the median and lateral atlantoaxial joints are present in the 70 mm fetus (Fig. 5-9). Synovial folds contain numerous collagenous fibers and blood vessels in the 170 mm fetus (Fig. 5-13).

Cartilage canals of the axis are first seen in the body in the 60 mm fetus (Fig. 5-8), and in the dens in the 90 mm fetus (Fig. 5-10). The ossification centers, one in the body and two in the dens, are first seen in the axis of the 120 mm fetus (Fig. 5-11). The paired ossification centers of the dens are fused by the 200 mm fetus (Fig. 5-14). A double-sided cartilaginous plate between the body and dens of the axis is formed in the 260mm fetus (Figs. 5-15 and 5-16), and remain until birth along with the longitudinal growing portion of the body and dens of the axis (Figs. 5-17 and 5-18).

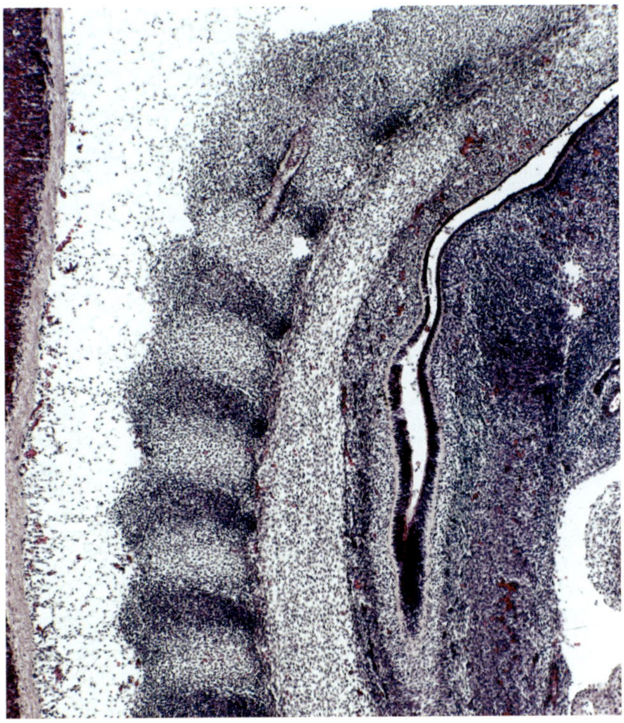

Fig. 5-1. Sagittal section, 14 mm, stage 18 embryo, showing the condensation of sclerotomal cells around the notochord. The basilar part of occipital segments, upper cervical notochord, and primordia of upper cervical vertebrae are shown.

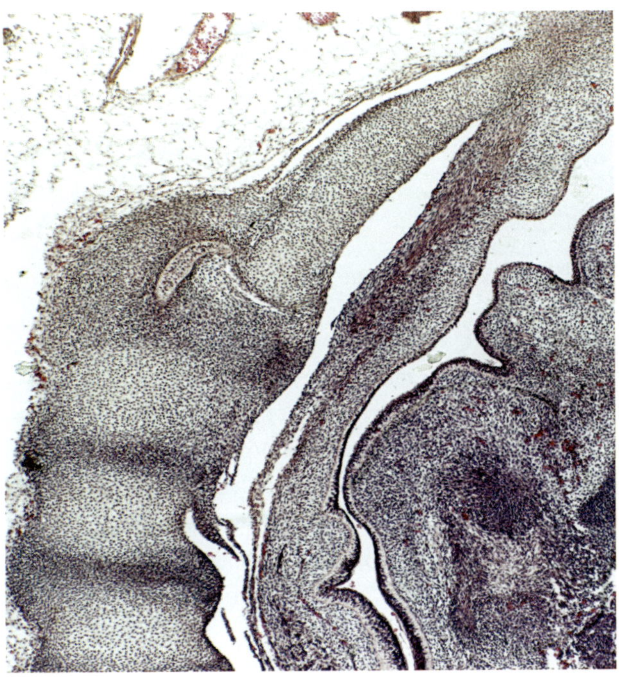

Fig. 5-2. Sagittal section through the part of the occipitocervical region of a 15 mm, stage 18 embryo, showing basispheniod and definitive cervical vertebrae.

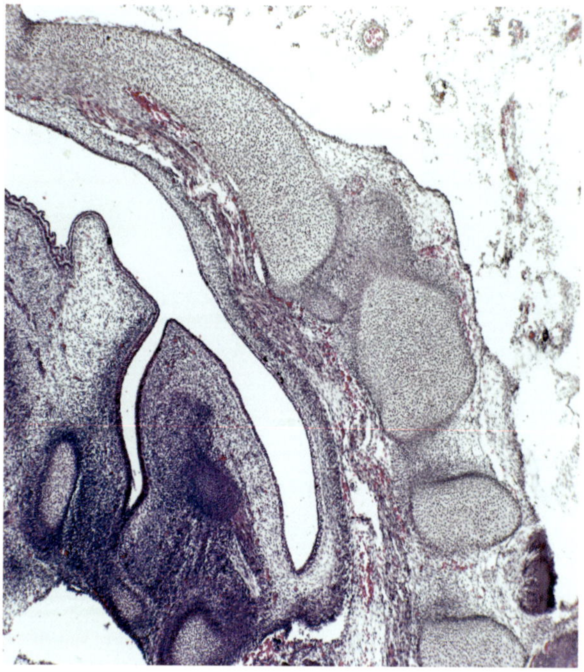

Fig. 5-3. Sagittal section through part of the occipitocervical region in a 24 mm, stage 21 embryo to show fusion of cartilaginous atlas and axis. The basilar part of occipital segments and the ventral arch of the atlas are seen.

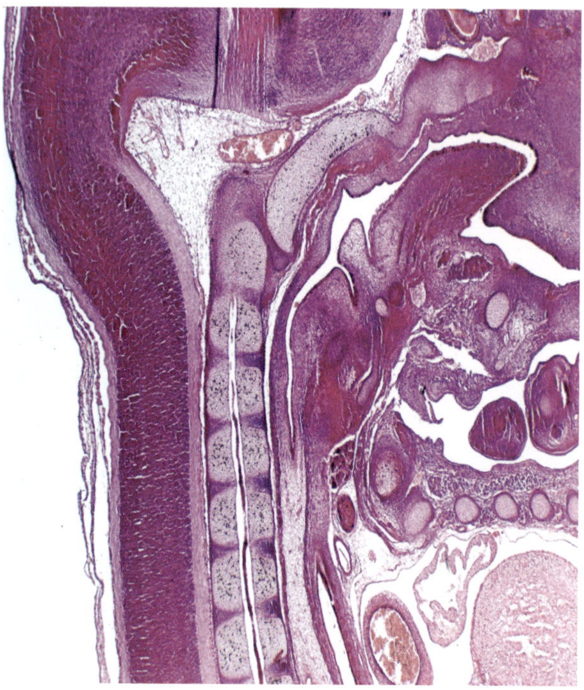

Fig. 5-4. Sagittal section through the midline of the vertebral body in a 24 mm, stage 21 embryo, showing the notochord and cartilaginous centrum. The chondrified ventral arches of the atlas and axis as well as the bodies of the third-seventh cervical vertebrae are seen. Fusion of the atlas and axis is also seen.

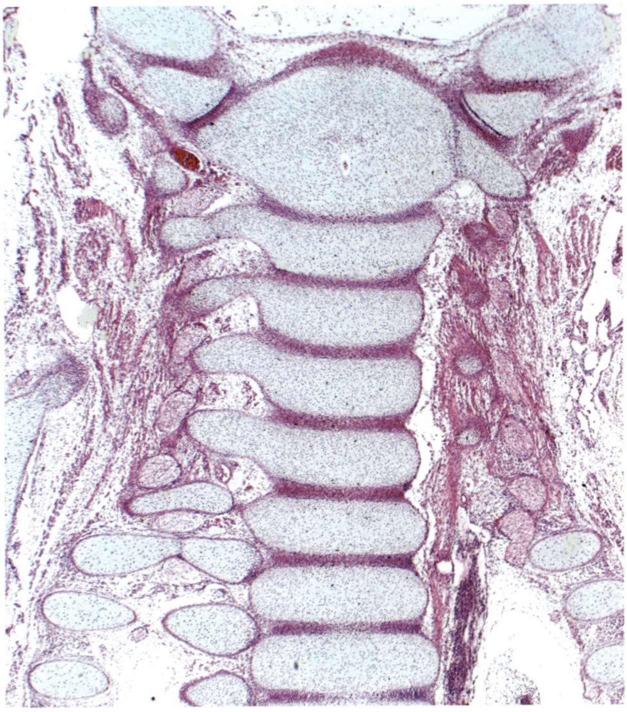

Fig. 5-5. Frontal section, 25 mm, stage 22 embryo, showing the basisphenoid, arches of the atlas, axis, and the third-seventh cervical vertebrae. The homogenous interzones in the atlanto-occipital and atlanto-axial joints are shown. A single cartilage anlage, including the body and both transverse processes, is clearly seen at the level third to sixth cervical vertebrae.

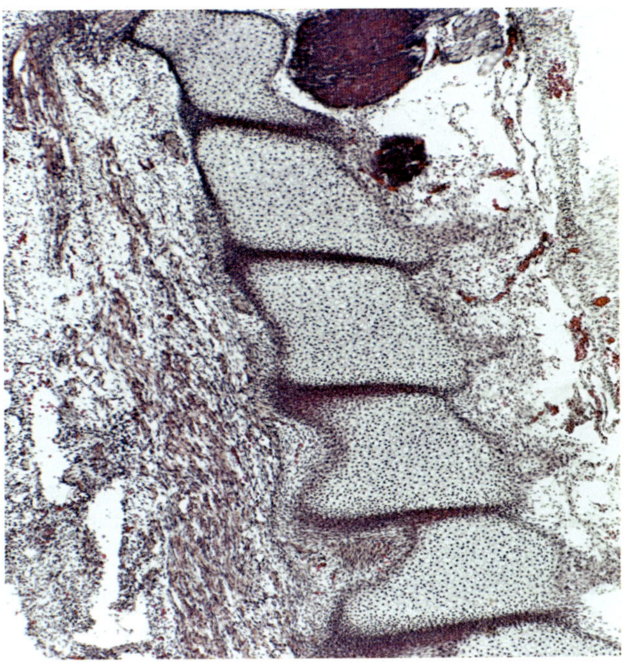

Fig. 5-6. Sagittal section through the part of the cervical region from a 25 mm embryo, showing cartilaginous centrum and intervertebral disc of the third-seventh cervical vertebrae.

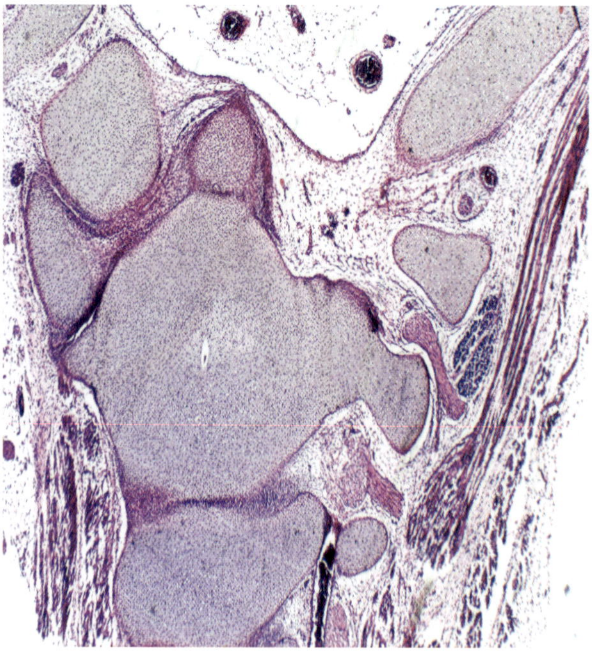

Fig. 5-7. Frontal section through part of the occipitocervical region of a 30 mm fetus to show the beginning cavitation of early atlanto-occipital and atlanto-axial joints. The tip of the dens and the body of the axis are shown. The atlanto-occipital membrane, alar ligament, and atlanto-axial ligament are well demonstrated.

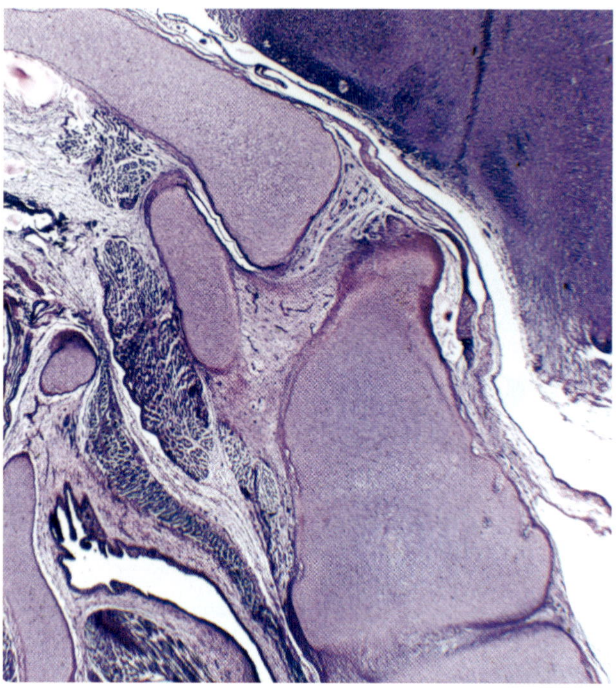

Fig. 5-8. Sagittal section through part of the occipitocervical region in a 60 mm fetus to show the dens, the body of the axis, the anterior arch of the atlas and part of the occiput. The transverse ligament of the atlas and apical ligament of the dens are seen. The tectorial membrana is also seen. The synovial joint between the transverse ligament of the atlas and the dens is observed. Cartilage canals in the dens are first seen.

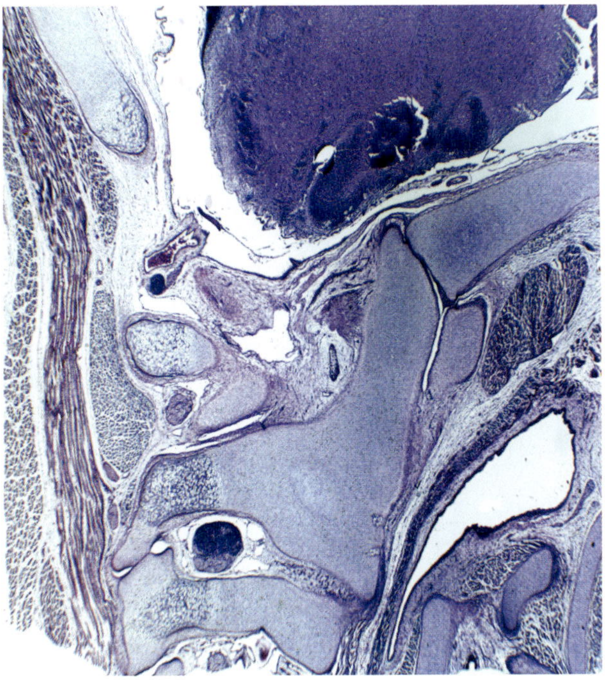

Fig. 5-9. Sagittal section through part of the occipitocervical region of a 70 mm fetus to show progressing ossification of the vertebral arch. The synovial joint between the transverse ligament of the atlas and dens is observed. Note the spinal ganglia in the intervertebral foramina. Cartilage canals in the dens and body are also seen.

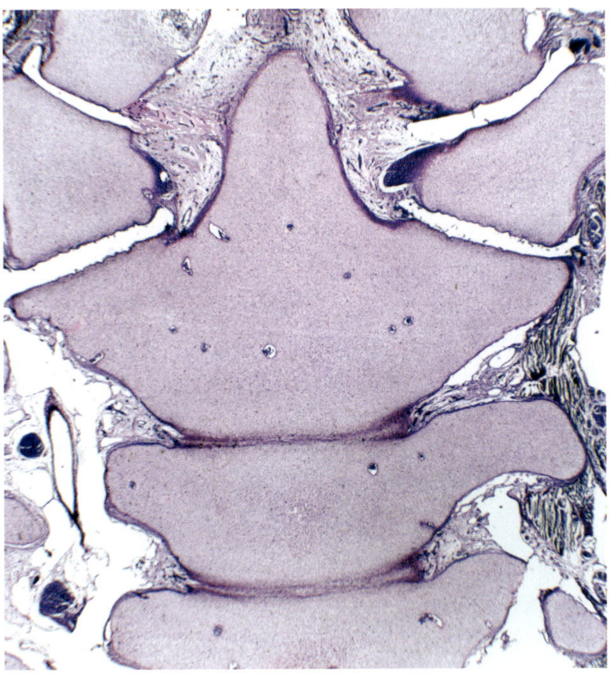

Fig. 5-10. Frontal section through part of the occipitocervical region of a 90 mm fetus to show atlanto-occipital and lateral atlantoaxial joints. The alar ligament is attached to the side of the dens and to the medial side of the condyle of the occipital bone. Cartilage canals in first-fourth cervical vertebrae are seen.

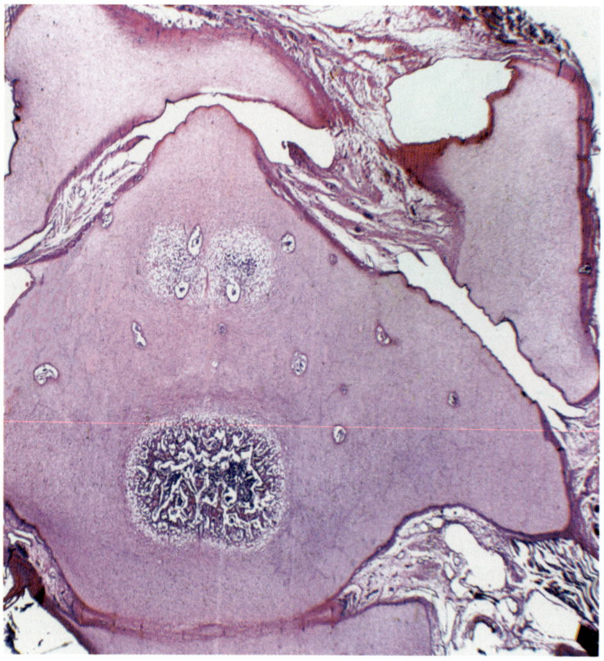

Fig. 5-11. Frontal section through the axis of a 120 mm fetus to show three ossification centers, one in the body and a paired center in the dens.

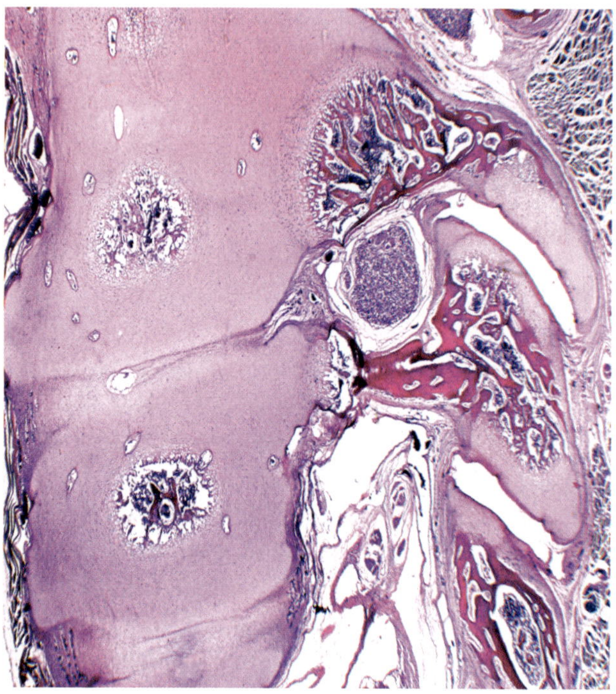

Fig. 5-12. Sagittal section through part of second-third cervical vertebrae of a 140 mm fetus to show progression of endochondral ossification of the bodies and vertebral arches. The spinal ganglia in the intervertebral foramina are shown.

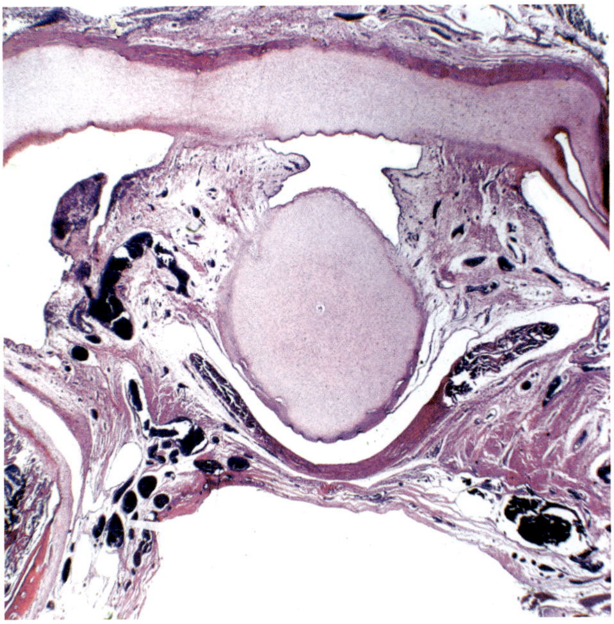

Fig. 5-13. Transverse section through part of the atlantoaxial joint from a 170 mm fetus to show the transverse ligament of the atlas. The median atlantoaxial joint contains two synovial cavites located between the dens and a ring formed by the anterior arch of the atlas and the transverse liament of the atlas. The synovial folds contain numerous collagenous fibers and blood vessels.

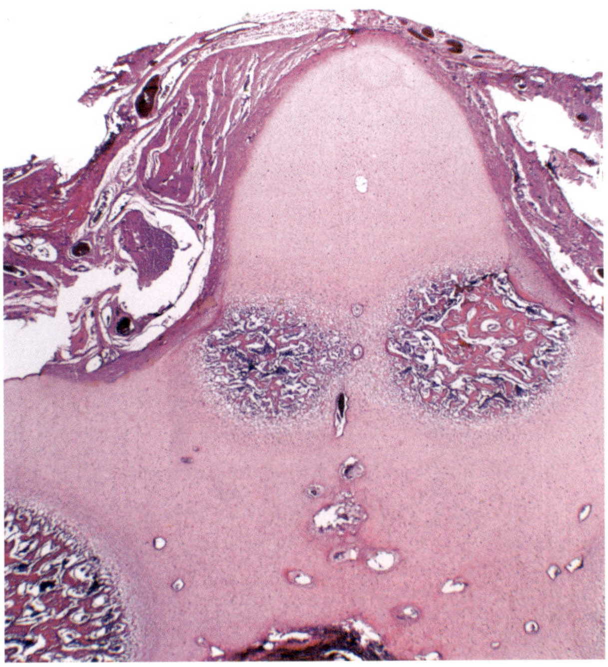

Fig. 5-14. Frontal section through part of the axis in a 200 mm fetus to show endochondral ossification. Two adjacent zones of ossifiction of the dens and body are shown.

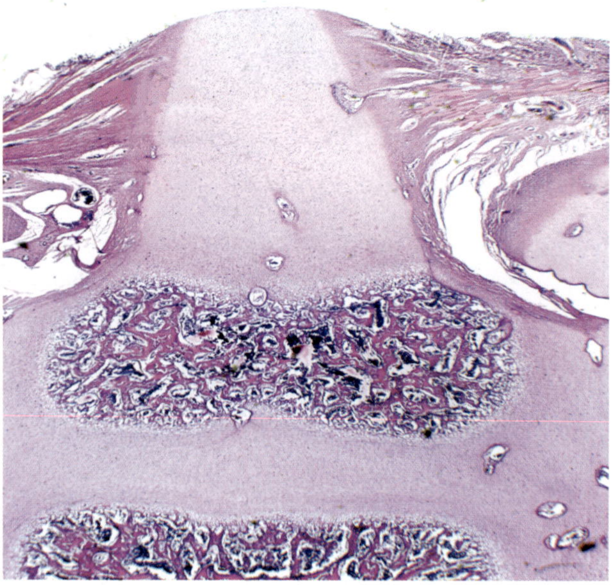

Fig. 5-15. Frontal section through part of the axis from a 260 mm fetus, showing endochondral ossification of the dens and body. Two adjacent zones of endochondral ossification of the body and dens are shown. Note the alar ligament.

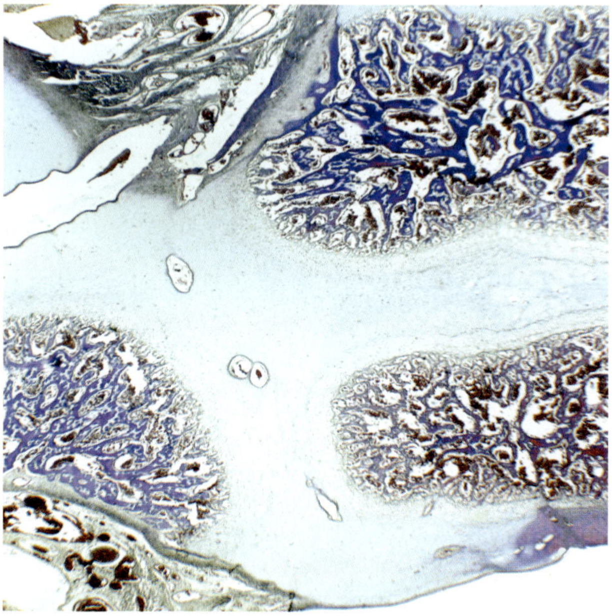

Fig. 5-16. Frontal section through part of the axis from a 260 mm fetus to show endochondral ossification. Endochondral ossification and its association with cartilage canals of the dens and body are seen.

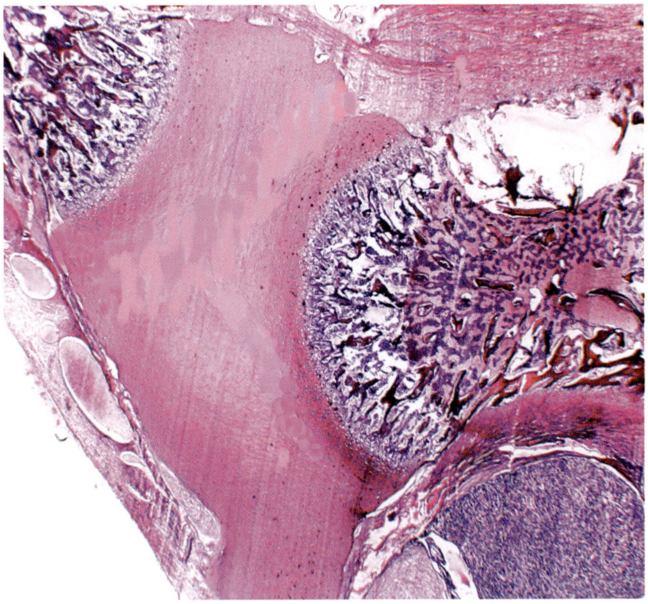

Fig. 5-17. Transverse section through part of the cervical vertebra in a 280 mm fetus to show the progressing ossification of a vertebral body and neural arch. Note the anterior longitudinal ligament and spinal ganglion.

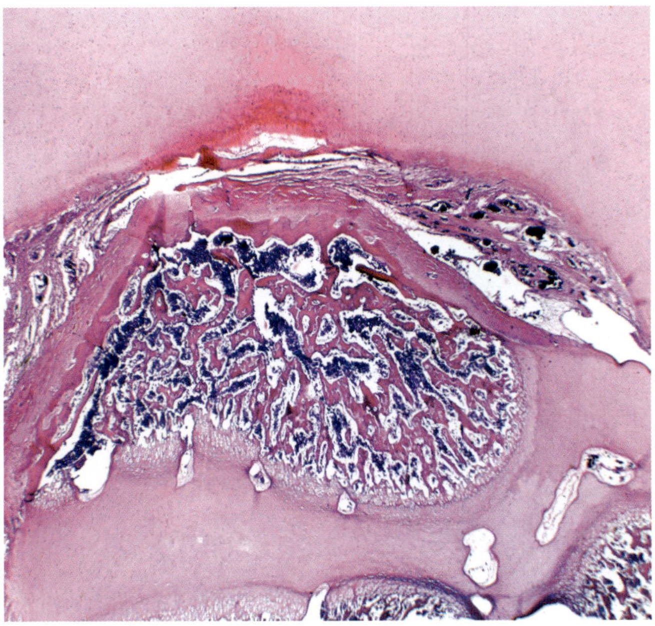

Fig. 5-18. Frontal section through part of the occipitocervical region in a 280 mm fetus to show ligaments connecting the axis with the occipital bone. Ossification of the dens and body of the axis has reached its anterior and posterior wall.

References

Bardeen CR: Early development of the cervical vertebrae and the base of the occipital bone in man. *Am J Anat* 8: 181-186, 1908.

Jenkins FA: The evolution and development of the dens of the mammalian axis. *Anat Rec* 164: 173-184, 1969.

Kim HK: The prenatal development of the dens in human fetuses. *Korean J Anat* 9: 69-77, 1976.

O'Rahilly R, Muller E, Meyer DB: The human vertebral column at the end of the embryonic period proper. The occipitocervical region. *J Anat* 136: 181-195, 1983.

Peacock A: Observations on the prenatal development of the intervertebral disc in man. *J Anat* 85: 260-274, 1951.

Sensenig EC: The development of the occipital and cervical segments and their associated structure in human embryos. *Contrib Embryol Carnegie Inst* 36: 141-152, 1957.

The Development of the Thoracic Vertebrae

Chapter 06

The primordium of the vertebral body, vertebral arch, transverse process, and the rib can be recognized to appear as a common blastemal mass from the 9 mm embryo and to complete the chondrification in the 22 mm embryo (Figs. 6-1, 6-2, and 6-3). By the time chondrification begins, the rib cartilage becomes separated from the vertebra by the development of primitive articulation of the head of the rib (Fig. 6-4). A pair of chondrification centers fuse across the midline to form the cartilaginous vertebral body. A similar chondrification center forms in each half of the neural arch and eventually extends dorsally to fuse behind the neural tube with its counterpart of the opposite side. The spinous and transverse processes develop from extensions of chondrification centers in the vertebral arch (Figs. 6-5 and 6-6).

In a 23 mm fetus, the homogenous interzone of articulation of the head of the rib appears and is divided into a three-layered interzone in the 30 mm fetus (Fig. 6-5). Primitive joint cavities of the articulation of the head of the rib and costovertebral joints are present around the periphery of the joint in the 35 mm and 50 mm fetuses, respectively (Figs. 6-8 and 6-9). In a 45 mm fetus, endochondral ossification in the rib has begun. As endochondral ossification proceeds ventrally and dorsally, growth zones become established in a 160 mm fetus (Fig. 6-17).

The ossification centers, one in each arch and one in the body, are first seen in the vertebrae. Usually endochondral ossification is more advanced in the pedicles than in the body (Fig. 6-11). By the 80 mm fetus, a large number of ossification centers are present simultaneously in the thoracic vertebrae, and as the fetal month proceeds, ossification is gradually extended to the cervical and sacral vertebrae (Figs. 6-14, 6-16, 6-18, and 6-20).

The cartilage canals of the thoracic vertebrae are first observed in the 60 mm fetus (Fig. 6-10). Cartilage canals are identified as vascular channels arising from perichondrium surfaces. A number of cartilage canals are observed around the primary center of ossification in the 70 mm fetus (Fig. 6-12). The canals are eventually eroded from the main medullary cavity and remain at only peripheral regions of growth cartilage. Cartilaginous plates make their appearance on the cranial and dorsal surfaces of the vertebral body in the 280 mm fetus and remain until birth as the longitudinal growing portion of the vertebrae.

By the 7 mm embryo, mesenchymal tissue, derived from the denser portion of the vertebral primordium, condenses into an intervertebral disc within each interspace. The anulus fibrosus is noted as densely arranged cells about each pole of the sclerotome. The concentric fibers of the anulus fibrosus appear in the 23 mm embryo and are composed of lamina of fibrous tissue, fibrocartilage, and loosely arranged cells in the 220 mm fetus. Throughout the fetal life, the outermost anulus fibrosus and layer of fibrocartilage in the ventral portion are much more compact than those the dorsal. Nucleus pulposus derived from the notochord consists of round cells surrounded by a fibrous ring in the 32 mm fetus (Fig. 6-7). Nucleus pulposus is an oval mucoid substance occupying the central portion of the intervertebral disc, being nearer to the posterior than to the anterior border of the anulus fibrosus (Fig. 6-13). At term, nucleus pulposus is composed of chondrocyte-like cells, dispersed within an intercellular matrix in which there is a loose network of notochordal cells.

The primitive joint cavity of the zygapophyseal joint is present around the periphery of the joint in the 60 mm fetus (Fig. 6-10) and complete in the 70 mm fetus (Fig. 6-12). Synovial tissue in the zygapophyseal joint is observed in the 130 mm fetus (Fig. 6-15).

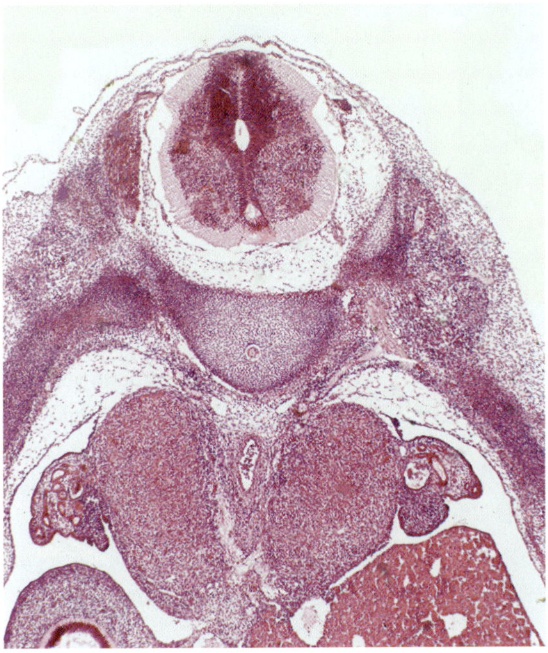

Fig. 6-1. Transverse section through the spinal cord region in a 14 mm, stage 18 embryo to show the vertebral body and ribs. The cartilaginous anlages of the vertebral body and rib are separated from the bodies by loose connective tissue. The pedicles and body are formed.

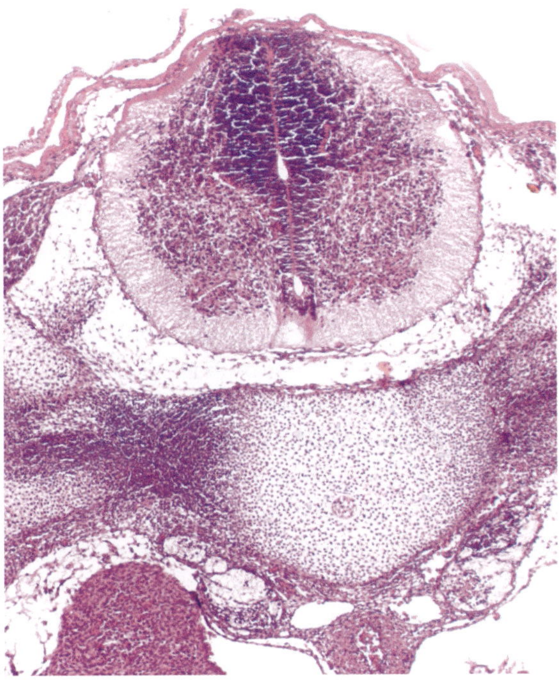

Fig. 6-2. Tranverse section through part of thoracic vertebra of a 22 mm, stage 21 embryo, showing chondrification of the vertebral body and ribs. Articulation of the head of the rib appears in the homogenous interzone. Vertebral body and pedicle form a single cartilaginous model.

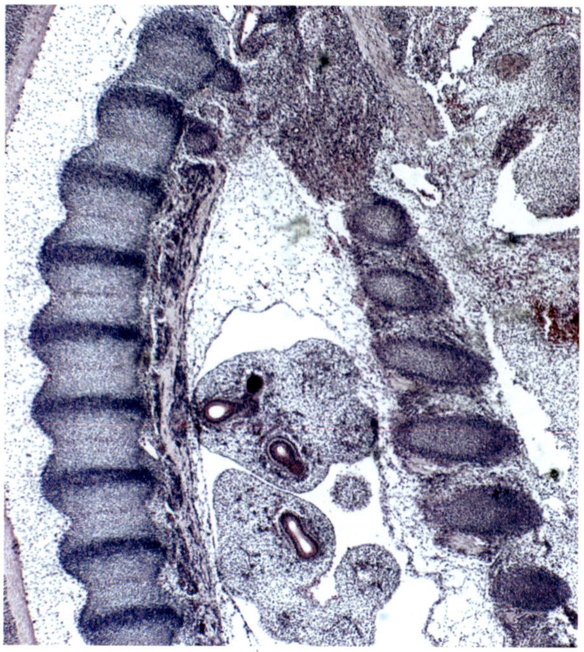

Fig. 6-3. Frontal section through part of the thoracic region from a 20 mm embryo, showing intervertebral disc and chondrified bodies. The densely packed mesenchymal cells constitute the intervertebral disc. Anterior to the lower part of the vertebrae the lung and ribs can be seen.

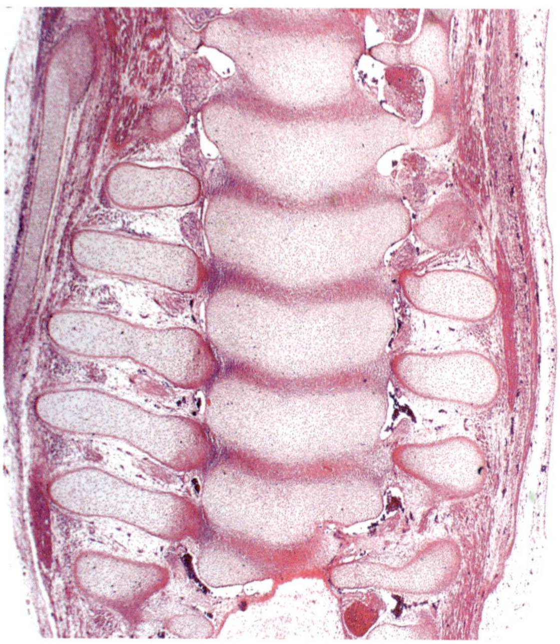

Fig. 6-4. Frontal section through part of the thoracic region from a 23 mm embryo, showing chondrified bodies and intervertebral discs. The anulus fibrosus is well formed. The interzone between the vertebral body and the head of the rib is in the early homogenous stage. The spinal ganglia are situated in the intervertebral foramina.

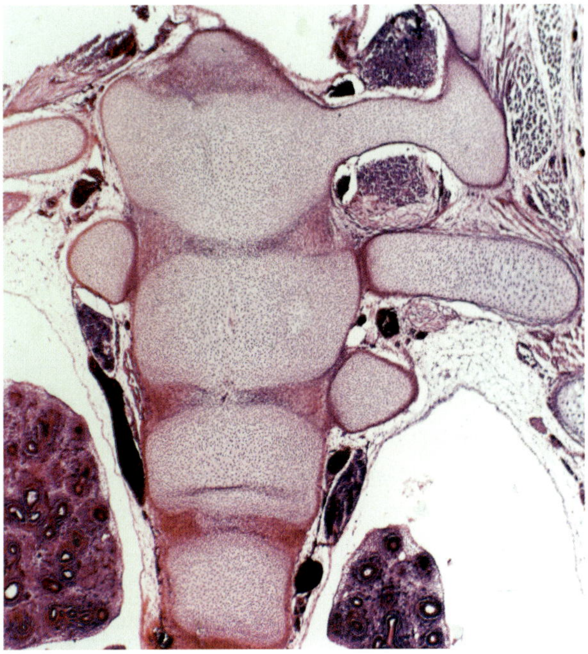

Fig. 6-5. Frontal section through thoracic region of a 30 mm fetus to show intervertebral discs and chondrified bodies. Articulation of the head of the rib appears as a three-layered interzone.

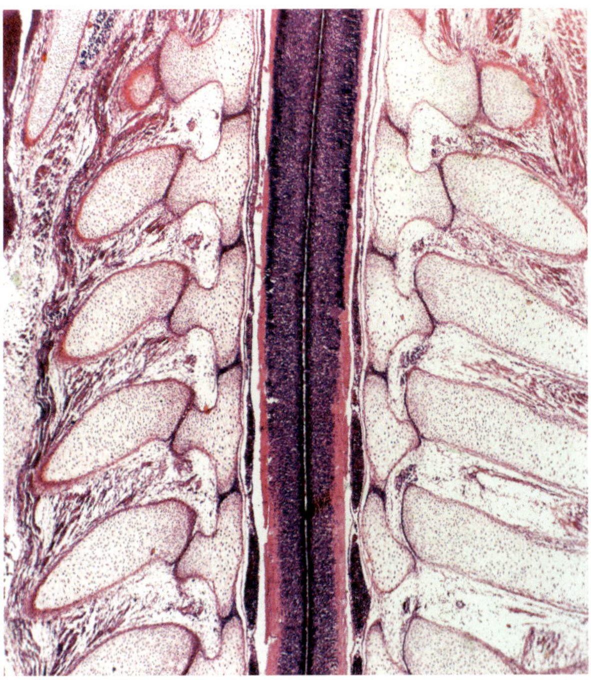

Fig. 6-6. Frontal section through part of the thoracic vertebrae of a 30 mm fetus, showing the three-layered interzone of the zygapophyseal and costotransverse joints.

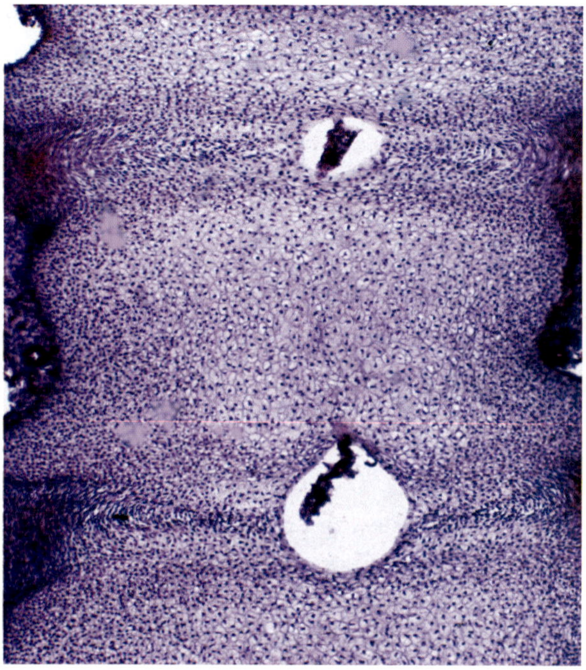

Fig. 6-7. Sagittal section through part of the thoracic vertebrae of a 32 mm fetus, showing the notochord and intervertebral disc. The notochord is degenerating except in the region of the intervertebral disc, where it persists as the nucleus pulposus. The anulus fibrosus is well formed.

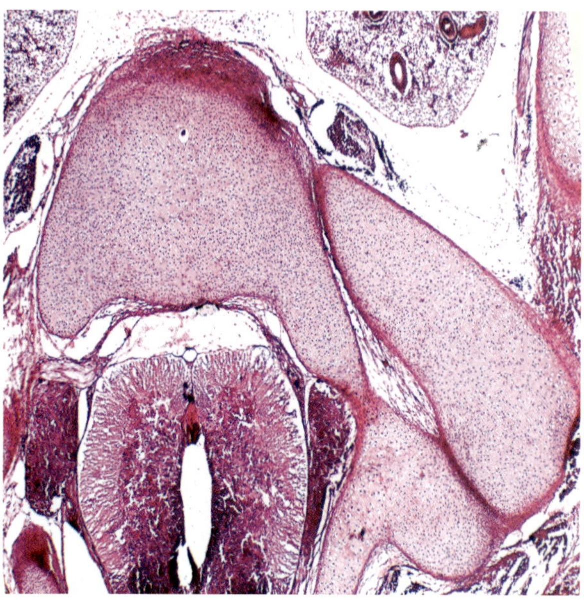

Fig. 6-8. Transverse section through part of the thoracic vertebrae of a 35 mm fetus to show peripheral cavitation of the articulation of the head of the rib.

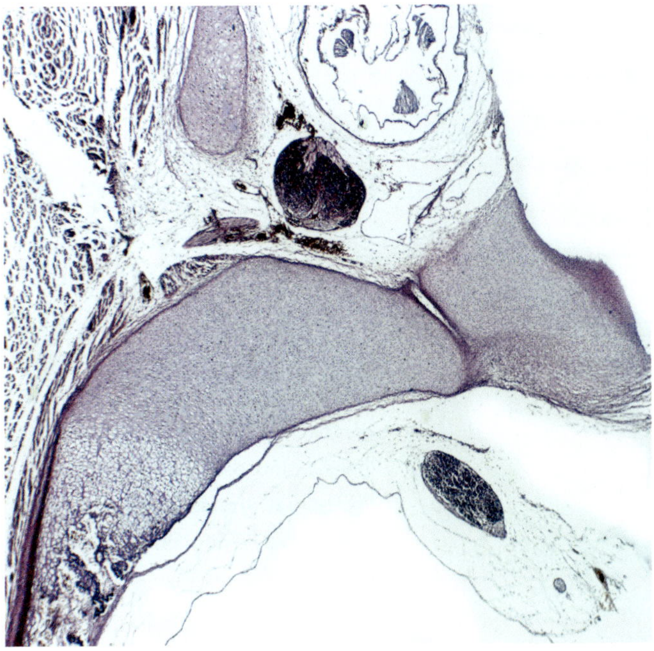

Fig. 6-9. Transverse section through part of the sixth rib in a 50 mm fetus, showing the ossification center of the rib. Endochondral ossification of the rib extends from the body to angle. Cavitation of articulation of the head of the rib is seen.

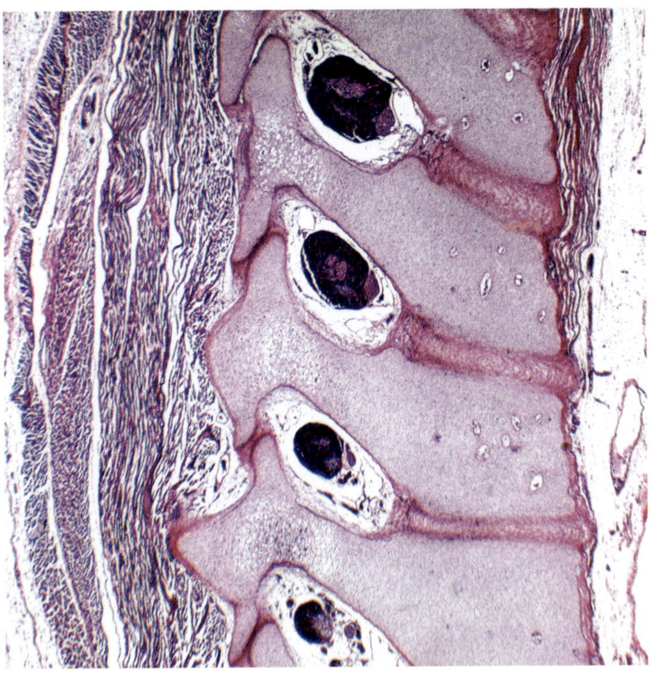

Fig. 6-10. Sagittal section through part of the thoracic vertebrae of a 60 mm fetus to show cartilage canals in the vertebral bodies. Cavitation of the zygapophyseal joint is seen. The spinal ganglia in intervertebral foramina are observed. Cartilage canals in the bodies of the vertebrae are seen.

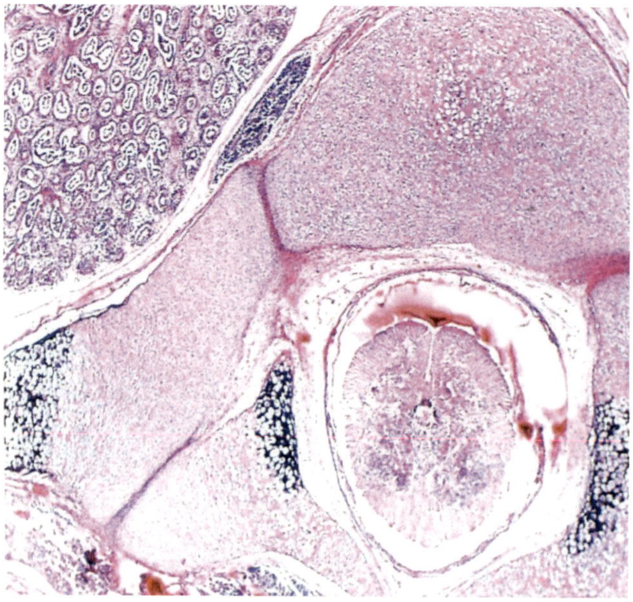

Fig. 6-11. Transverse section crosses the vertebral column of a 60 mm fetus to show ossification centers in the neural arch and rib. Ossification centers are visible in the neural arches and head of the rib but not in the body of the vertebra.

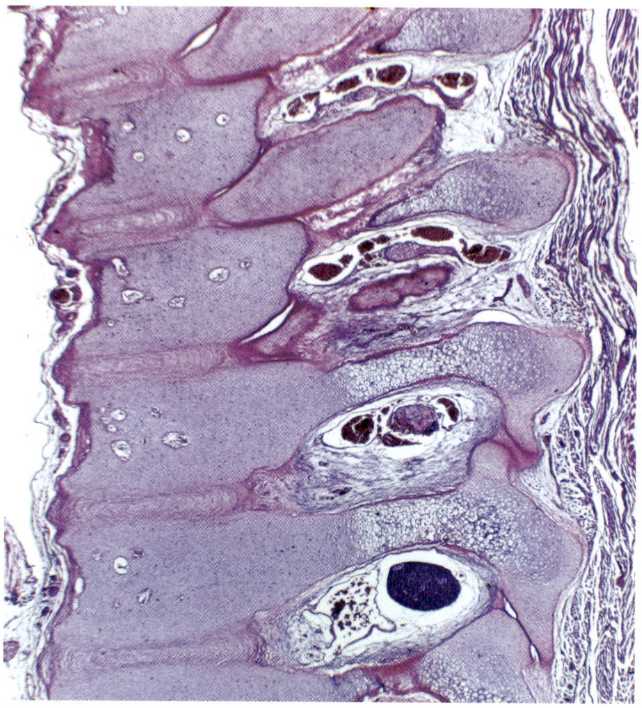

Fig. 6-12. Sagittal section through part of the thoracic vertebae from a 80 mm fetus to show cavitation in articulation of the head of the rib. Ossification center of the pars interarticularis is seen. There are numerous cartilage canals in the vertebral bodies. Note the zygapophyseal joint.

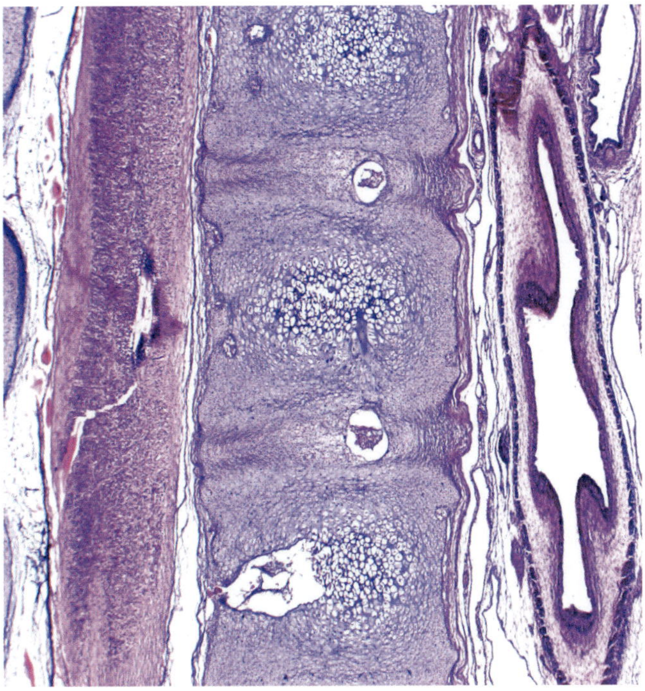

Fig. 6-13. Sagittal section through part of the thoracic vertebrae from a 80 mm fetus to show vertebral body having its ossification center and intervertebral disc exhibiting more or less a lamellar arrangement of different cell types. The spaces with notochordal cells extend posteriorly beyond the intermediate layer of the anulus fibrosus.

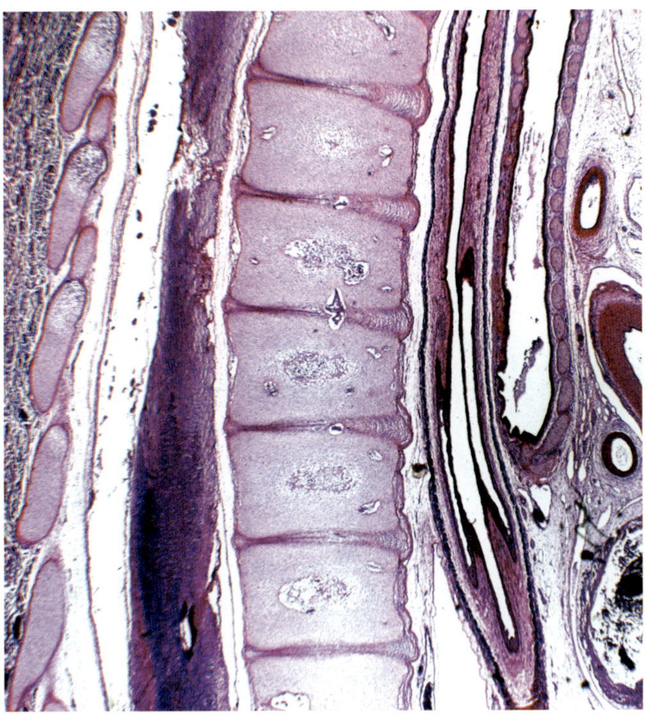

Fig. 6-14. Sagittal section through part of the thoracic vertebrae from a 100 mm fetus to show the ossification center in the bodies and neural arches of the vertebrae. Endochondral ossification in the bodies and its association with cartilage canals are seen. The proliferating notochordal cells and orderly arranged cells of different types of anulus fibrosus are seen.

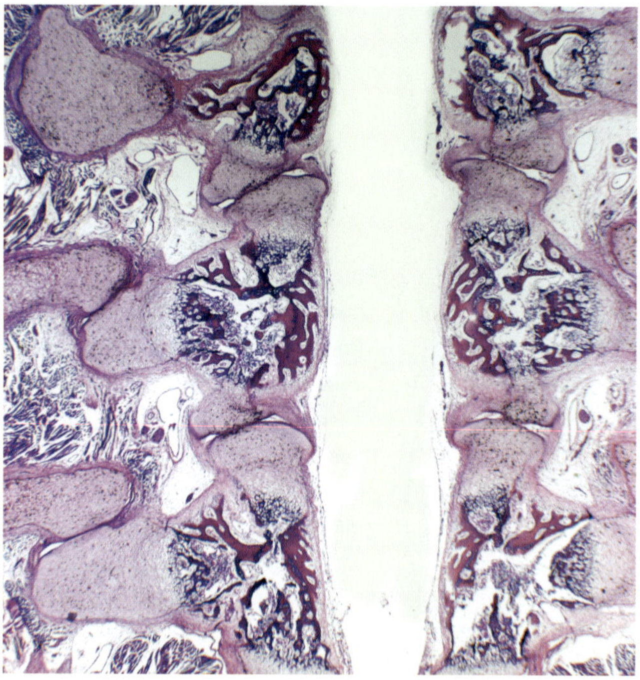

Fig. 6-15. Sagittal section through part of the thoracic vertebrae of a 130 mm fetus to show the zygapophysial and costotransverse joints. Endochondral ossification of the body has reached its pars interarticularis. Cavitations of the zygapophyseal and costotransverse joints are observed.

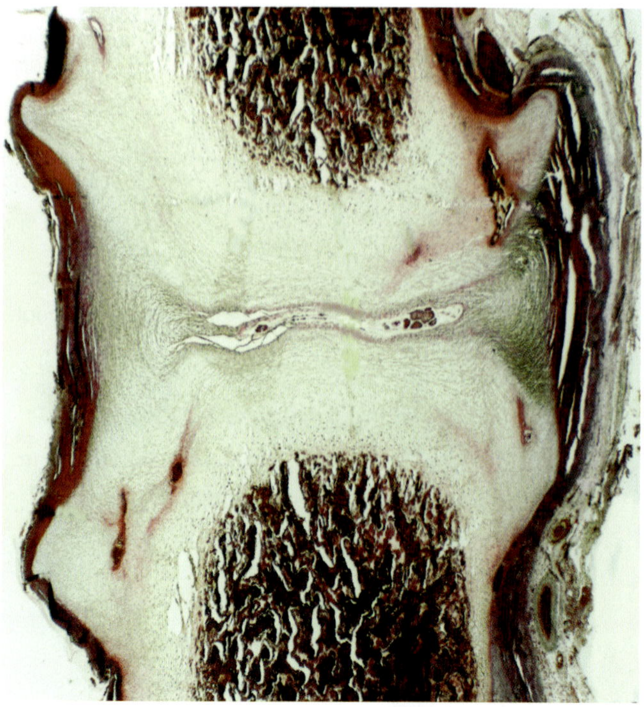

Fig. 6-16. Frontal section through part of the thoracic vertebrae of a 160 mm fetus, showing endochondral ossification of the vertebral body. The nucleus pulposus is an oval gelatinous mass which occupies the central portion of the disc. The anulus fibrosus is composed of layers of collagenous fibers.

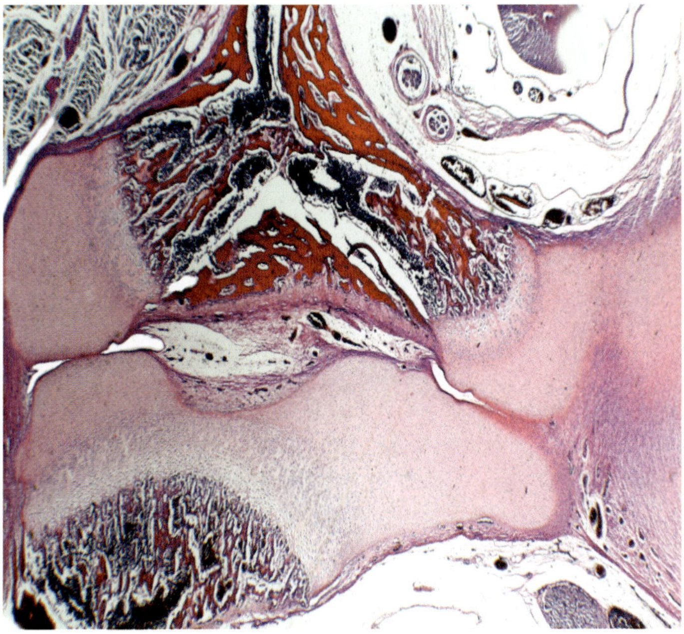

Fig. 6-17. Transverse section through part of the thoracic vertebrae from a the 160 mm fetus to show the ossification center in the neural arch. The ossification center of the rib extends from body to angle. Articulation of the head of the rib and costotransverse joint are clearly visible.

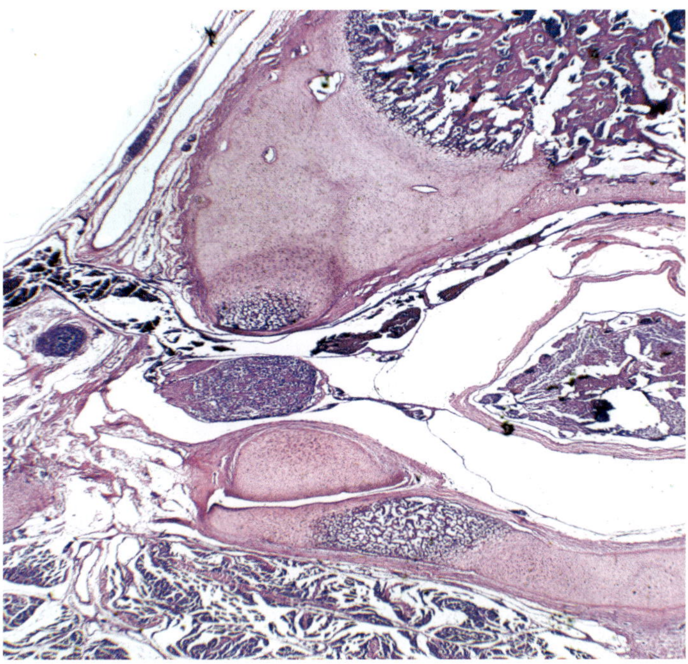

Fig. 6-18. Transverse section through part of the thoracic vertebrae from a 200 mm fetus to show the progressing ossification of a vertebral body. Endochondral ossification of the body has reached its anterior wall. Cavitation of the zygapophyseal joint is seen. Spinal ganglion and nerve root occupy the intervertebral foramen.

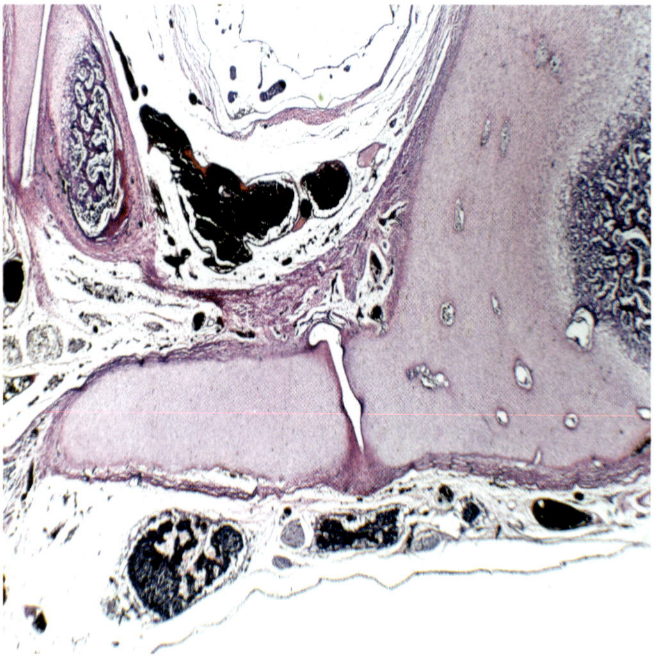

Fig. 6-19. Transverse section through part of the thoracic vertebrae from a 200 mm fetus, showing cartilage canals which are frequently seen near the ossification center of the vertebral body. Cavitation of articulation of the head of the rib is seen.

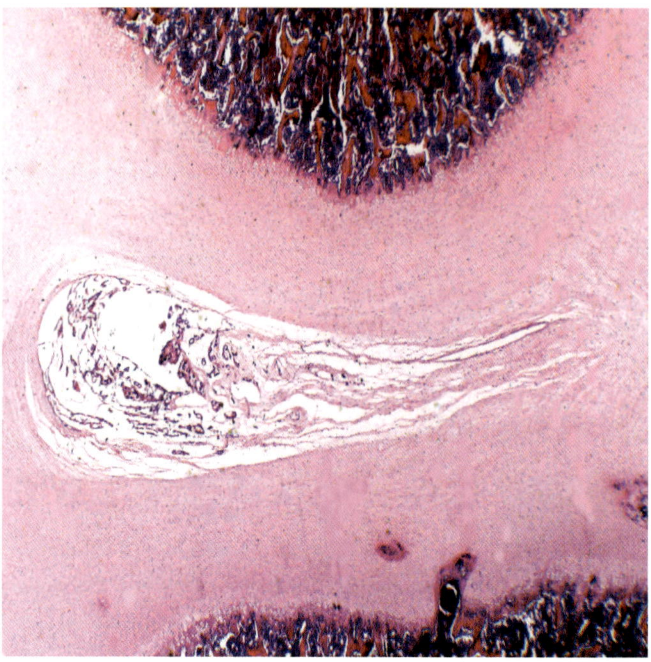

Fig. 6-20. Sagittal section through part of the thoracic vertebrae of a 220 mm fetus to show advanced stage of ossification. Note the typical columnar cartilaginous epiphyseal plate covering the cephalic and caudal surfaces of ossification. The matrix of the nucleus pulposus is arranged to form a loose network of poorly differentiated collagenous fiber. The anulus fibrosus is composed of layers of collagenous fibers.

References

Bardeen CR: The development of the thoracic vertebrae in man. *Am J Anat* 4: 163-174, 1905.

Coventry MB, Ghormley RK, Kernohan JW: The intervertebral disc: Its microscopic anatomy and pathology. *J Bone Joint Surg* 27A: 105-112, 1945.

Peacock A: Observation on the prenatal development of the intervertebral disc in man. *J Anat* 85: 260-274, 1951.

Yoon JR:. The prenatal development of the intervertebral disc in human fetuses and children. *Chonnam Medical J* 13: 219-234, 1976.

The Development of the Lumbar Vertebrae

Chapter 07

By the 15 mm embryo, the mesenchymal stage of the vertebral bodies and pedicles forms a single anlage (Figs. 7-1 and 7-2). Chondrification of the vertebral bodies and pedicles is completed by the 22 mm embryo (Fig. 7-3). The two centers in each centrum fuse across the midline to form a cartilaginous centrum in the 22 mm embryo (Fig. 7-4). Similar chondrification centers in the vertebral arches fuse with each other and the centrum in the 30 mm fetus (Fig. 7-6). The spinous and transverse processes develop from an extension of the chondrification centers in the vertebral arch (Figs. 7-7 and 7-8). The cartilage canals of the lumbar vertebrae are first observed in the 60 mm fetus. The ossification centers, one in the body and one in each half of the vertebral arch, are first seen in the vertebrae of the 70 mm fetus (Fig. 7-11). A number of ossification centers are present simultaneously in the thoracic and lumbar vertebral column of the 100 mm fetus (Fig. 7-12), and as the fetal month proceeds, ossification is gradually extended to the cervical and sacral vertebrae from thoracic and lumbar vertebrae (Fig. 7-16). Cartilage canals are observed around the primary center of ossification (Fig. 7-11). In the 120 mm fetus, cartilage canals of the bodies of vertebrae are abundant in the region, where the ossification is actively progressing (Fig. 7-14). Columns of cartilage cells make their appearance on the cranial and caudal to the center of ossification in the 240 mm fetus (Fig. 7-17) and remain until birth as the longitudinal growing portion of the vertebrae (Figs. 7-18 and 7-20). The processes of the bone formation in the vertebral bodies are found to possess morphological similarities to that occurring at the secondary center of the epiphysis of a long bone.

In the 15 mm embryo, mesenchymal tissue, derived from the denser portion of the vertebral primordium, condenses into an intervertebral disc within each interspace. The anulus fibrosus is noted as densely aggregated cells about each pole of the vertebrae in the 22 mm embryo (Fig. 7-4). In the 50 mm embryo, the concentric fibers of the anulus fibrosus are observed (Fig. 7-9) and are composed of lamina of fibrous tissue in the 100 mm fetus (Fig. 7-13). Throughout the fetal life, the outermost anulus fibrosus in the ventral portion is much more compact than that of the dorsal. Nucleus pulposus derived from the notochord consists of round cells surrounded by the anulus fibrosus in a 25 mm embryo (Fig. 7-5). In the 180 mm fetus, the nucleus pulposus is an oval gelatinous substance which occupies the central portion of the intervertebral disc, being nearer to the posterior than to the anterior border of the anulus fibrosus (Fig. 7-15). Viable and chondrocyte-like cells in nucleus pulposus exist in the specimen from the fetal age. During fetal life, the structure of notochordal cells and their persistance in the nucleus pulposus suggest that they may have a significant role in the formation and maintenance of the nucleus pulposus. In the youngest child, the nucleus pulposus is composed of the loose delicate fibrous strands embedded in a gelatinous matrix (Fig. 7-19).

In a 22 mm embryo, the anulus fibrosus is identifiable (Fig. 7-4). The anulus fibrosus, composed of layers of collagenous fibers, is firmly attached to the adjacent vertebrae in the 60 mm fetus (Fig. 7-10). By the 100 mm fetus, the fibers are directed obliquely between the vertebrae, and the fibers of innermost layers are perpendicular to each other (Fig. 7-13).

The anterior and posterior longitudinal ligaments appear as cellular condensation in the 20 to 25 mm embryos (Fig. 7-5). A few collagenous fibers are present in these structures by the 50 mm fetus, and by the 100 mm fetus the fibers form a dense collagenous framework (Figs. 7-11 and 7-13).

The caudal end of the spinal cord, situated at the caudal border of the coccygeal vertebrae at 8 weeks, reaches the level of the third lumbar vertebra at the end of the tenth month. The ventro-dorsal diameter of the lumbar enlargement is greater than that of the cervical on and after the fifth month. The lumbar enlargement extends from the tenth to twelfth thoracic vertebra during the entire fetal life.

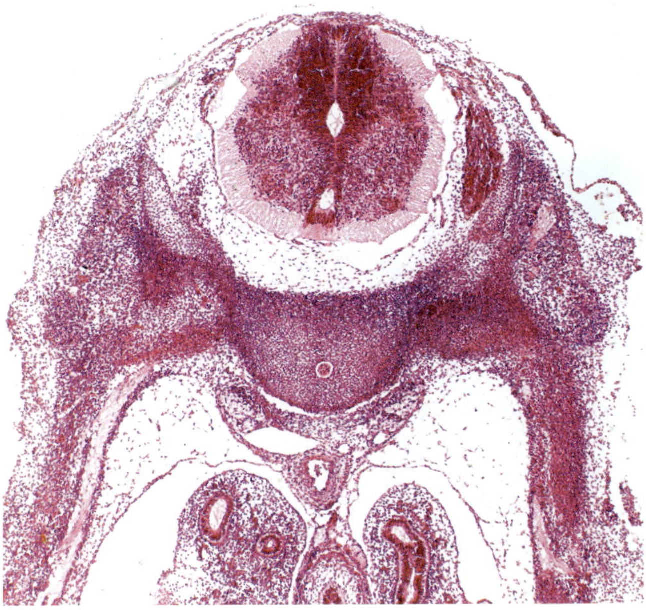

Fig. 7-1. Transverse section through part of the lumbar vertebrae in a 15 mm embryo, showing the vertebral body and spinal cord. The cartilaginous models of the vertebral body and pedicles are separated from body by loose connective tissue.

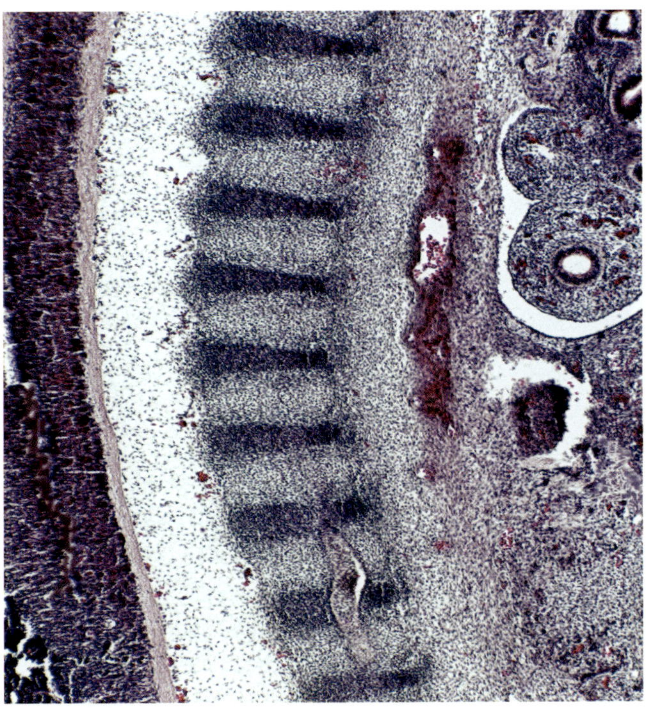

Fig. 7-2. Sagittal section through the midline of the vertebral body of a 15 mm embryo, showing the notochord and definitive vertebrae. The densely-packed mesenchymal cells constitute the intervertebral disc. Anterior to the caudal part of the vertebrae, the mesonephros can be seen.

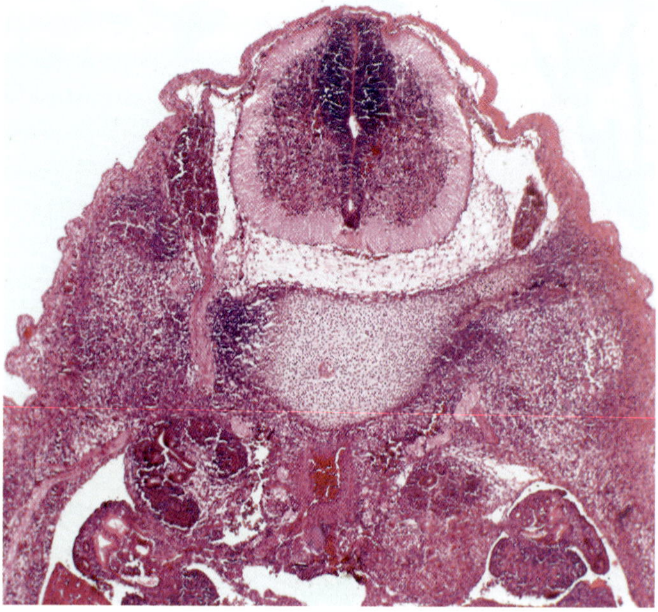

Fig. 7-3. Transverse section through the level of the second lumbar vertebra in a 22 mm embryo, showing chondrification of the vertebral body. The vertebral body and pedicles form a single cartilaginous model.

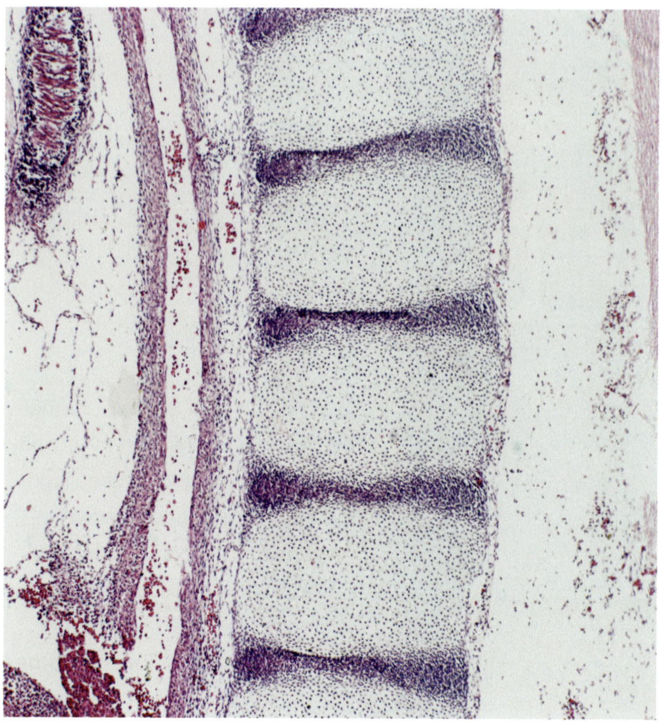

Fig. 7-4. Sagittal section through part of the lumbar vertebrae from a 22 mm embryo, showing the intervertebral discs and chondrified bodies. Anulus fibrosus is now identifiable.

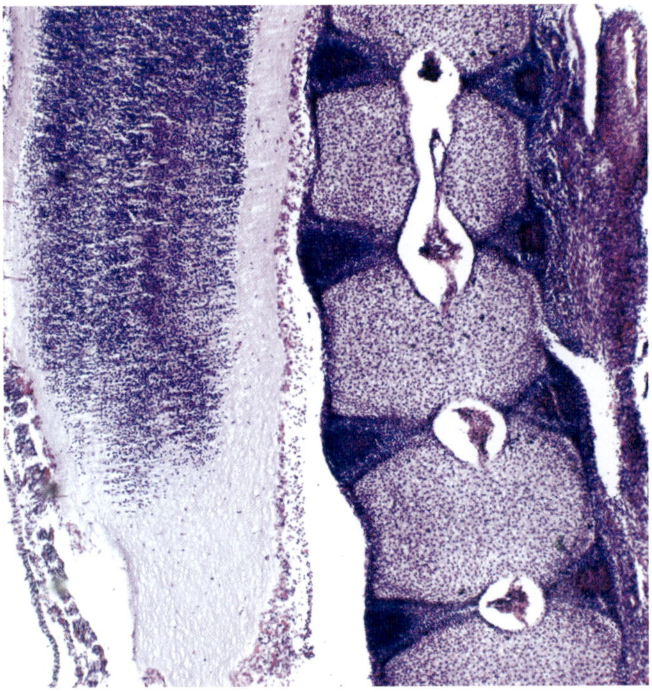

Fig. 7-5. Sagittal section through part of the lumbar vertebrae from a 25 mm embryo to show the intervertebral discs and chondrified bodies. Both the anterior and posterior longitudinal ligaments are seen. Remnants of the notochord, the future nucleus pulposus, are identifiable.

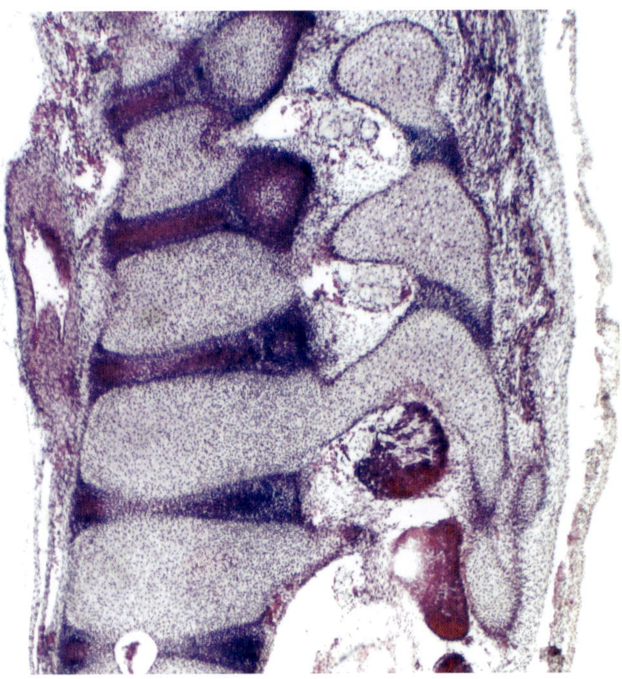

Fig. 7-6. Sagittal section through part of the lumbar vertebrae in a 30 mm fetus to show the cartilaginous vertebrae. The anulus fibrosus is now well formed. The articular interzone of the zygapophyseal joint appears as a homogenous structure.

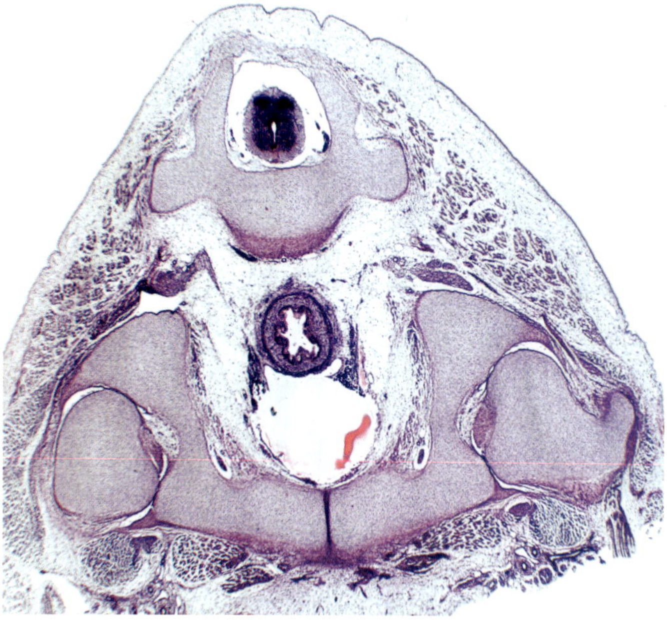

Fig. 7-7. Transverse section through part of fourth sacral vertebra in a 40 mm fetus to show spinal cord. The spinous process is not fused.

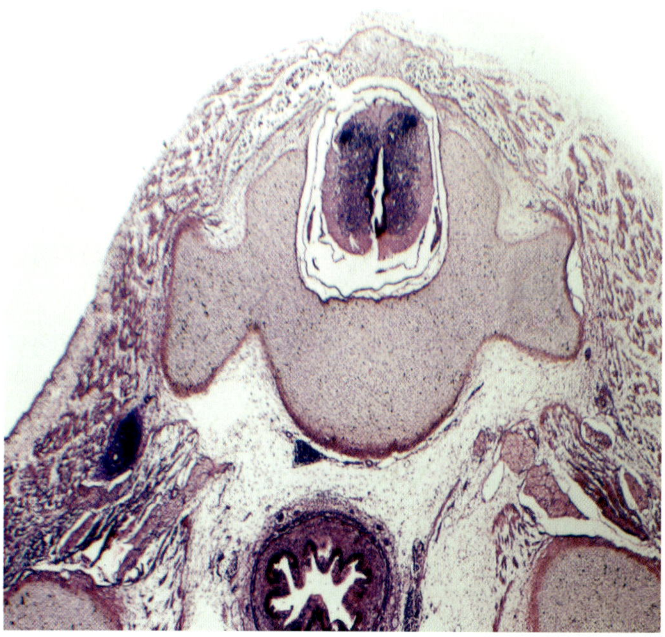

Fig. 7-8. Transverse section through the level of the third sacral vertebra in a 55 mm fetus to show the spinal cord and posterior elements. The posterior elements are still not fused. The spinal cord is well formed.

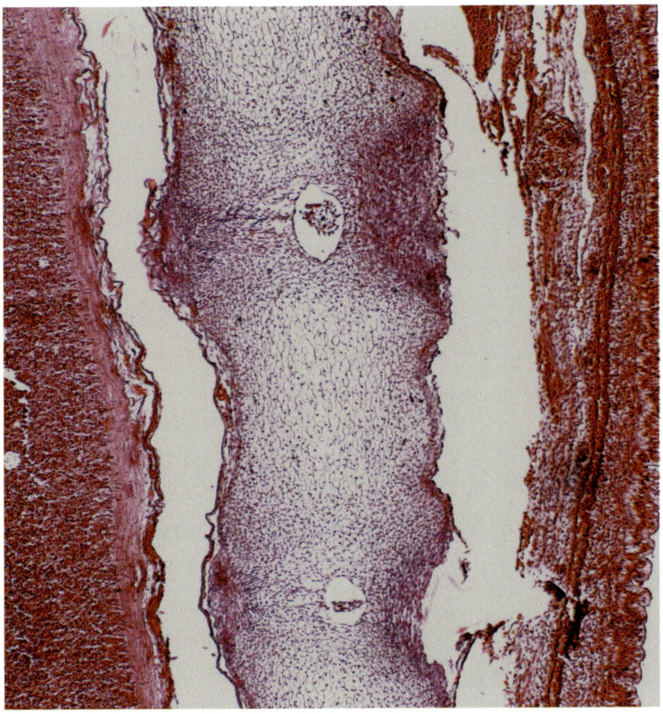

Fig. 7-9. Sagittal section through part of the lumbar vertebrae of a 50 mm fetus to show intervertebral disc. The hypertrophied chondrocytes are visible in the body. The anulus fibrosus exhibits more or less lamellar arrangement of different cell types.

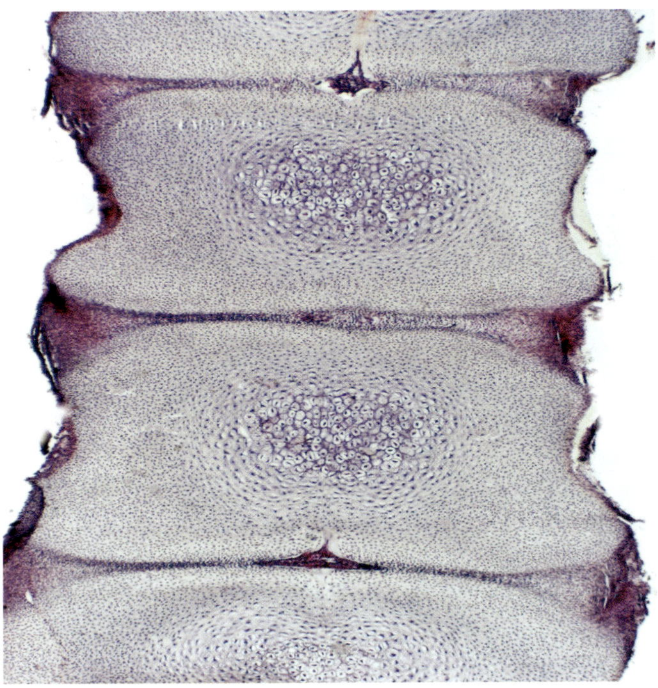

Fig. 7-10. Frontal section through part of the lumbar vertebrae of a 60 mm fetus to show the zone of hypertrophied cartilage cells. The anulus fibrosus and nucleus pulposus are seen. Remnants of the notochord in the body are also shown.

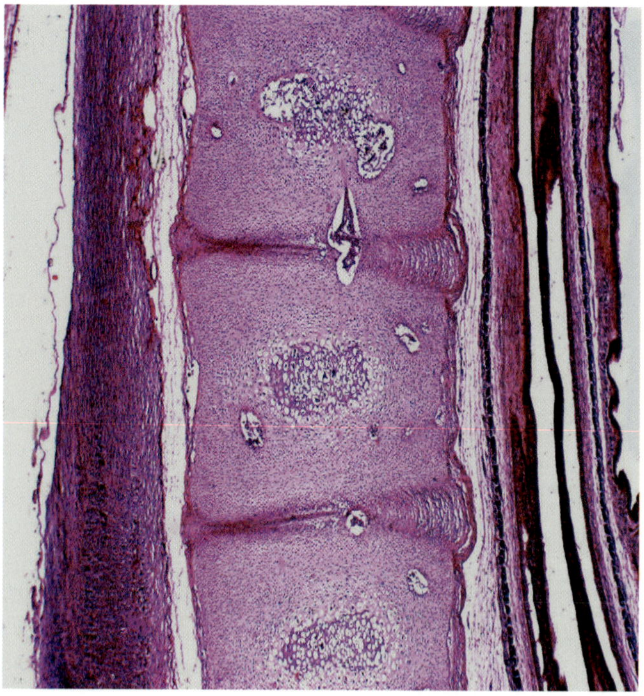

Fig. 7-11. Sagittal section through part of the lumbar vertebrae in a 70 mm fetus to show the primary centers of ossification in the vertebral bodies. Cartilage canals in the vertebral bodies are first seen. The anterior and the posterior longitudinal ligaments are seen. The anulus fibrosus and notochordal cells are observed.

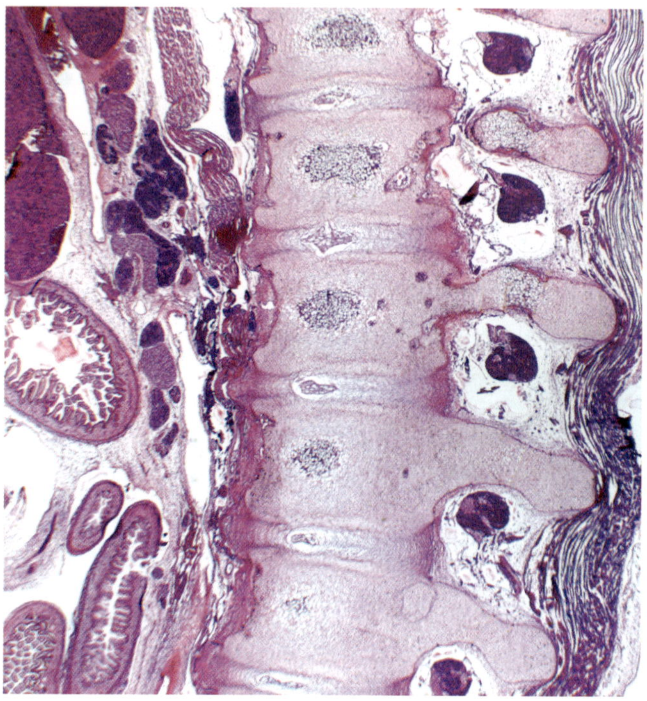

Fig. 7-12. Sagittal section through part of the lumbar vertebrae of a 100 mm fetus to show ossification centers. A large blood vessel enters from posterior surface. The notochordal cells and anulus fibrosus are well shown. The spinal ganglia are situated in the intervertebral foramina.

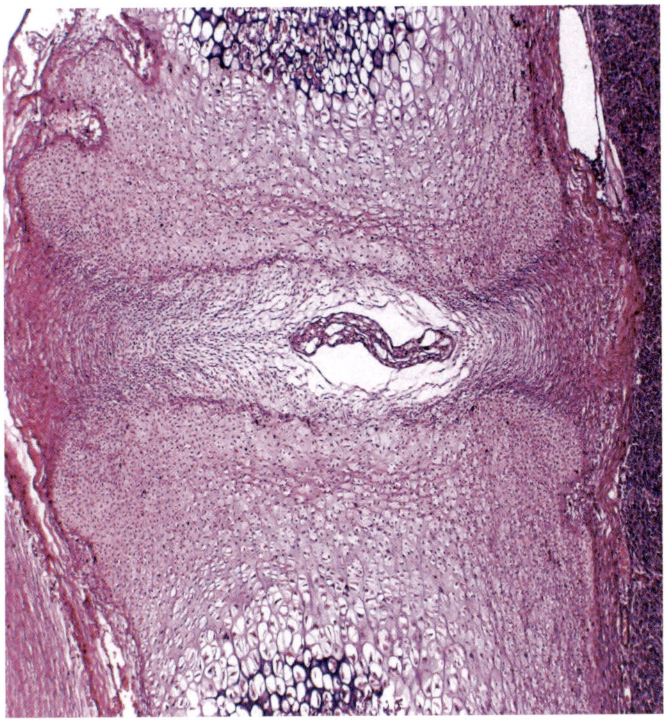

Fig. 7-13. Sagittal section from the specimen of a 100 mm fetus to show the vertebral body having its ossification centers and intervertebral disc. The nucleus pulposus and orderly-arranged cells of different types of anulus fibrosus are seen.

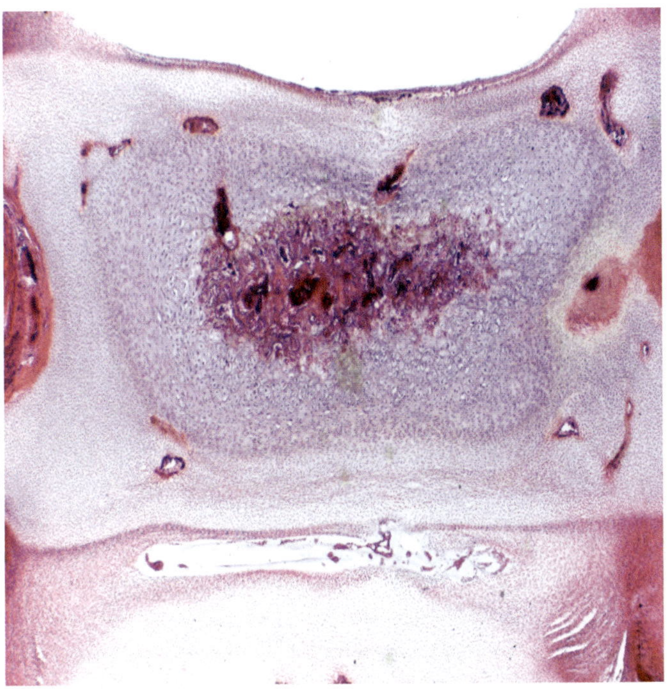

Fig. 7-14. Frontal section of the lumbar vertebrae of a 120 mm fetus to show endochondral ossification and its association with cartilage canals. Note the fragmentation of the notochordal cells and mucoid substance.

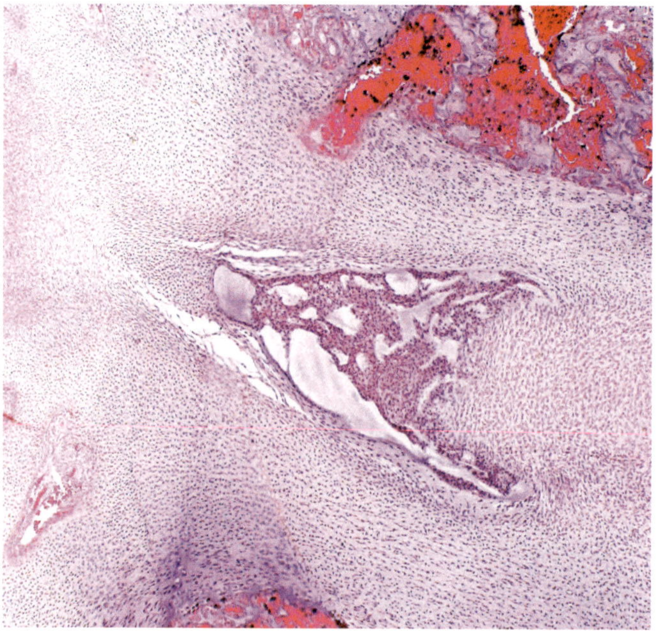

Fig. 7-15. Sagittal section from the specimen of a 180 mm fetus to show the intervertebral disc. The nucleus pulposus is an oval gelatinous mass which extends posteriorly beyond the intermediate layer of the anulus fibrosus.

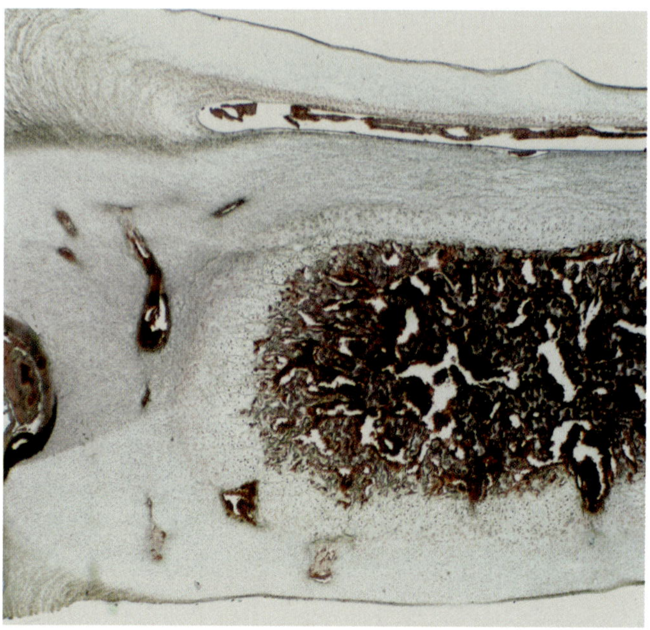

Fig. 7-16. Frontal section of a body of the lumbar vertebra in a 200 mm fetus to show endochondral ossification and the multitude of cartilage canals. The anulus fibrosus and fragmentation of the notochordal cells are clearly visible.

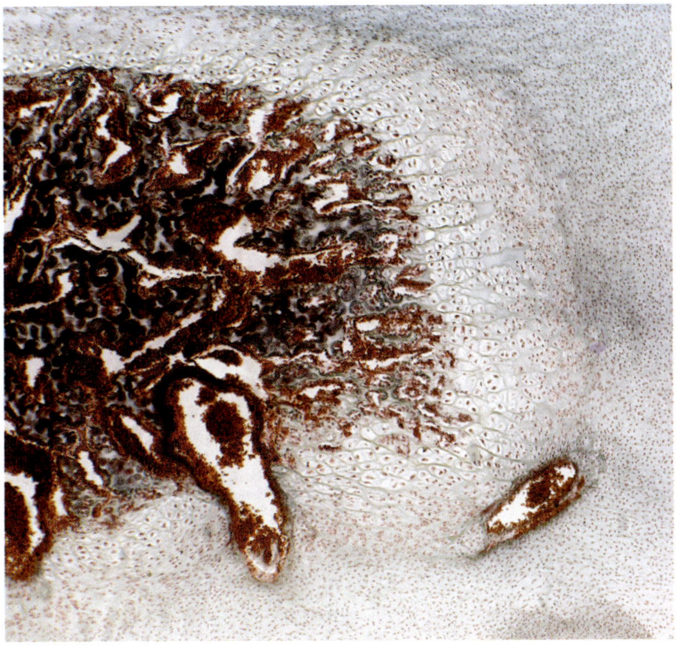

Fig. 7-17. Frontal section of a body of the lumbar vertebra in a 240 mm fetus to show the advanced stage of ossification. At this time, columnar cartilage first appears in the form of an epiphyseal plate across its cephalic and caudal surfaces.

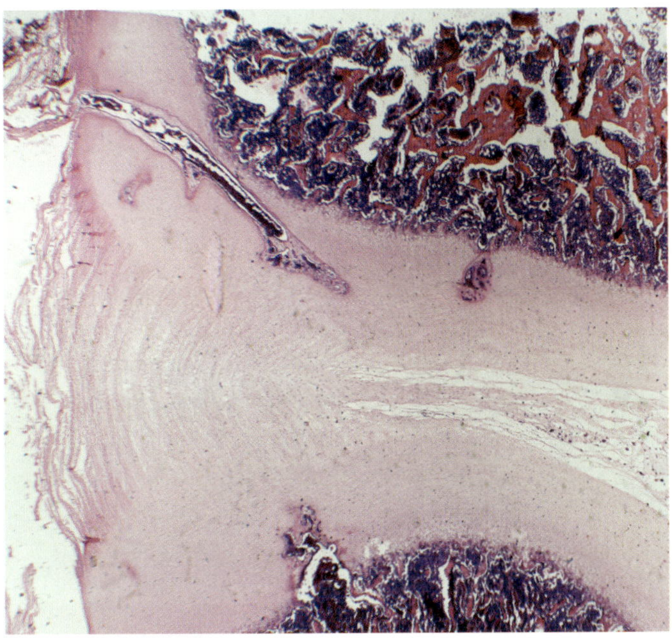

Fig. 7-18. Sagittal section of the bodies of the lumbar vertebrae in a 260 mm fetus to show endochondral trabeculae in the body. Ossification of the body has reached the entire depth of the vertebral body. Note a periosteal blood vessel communicates with the blind end of the superficial canal.

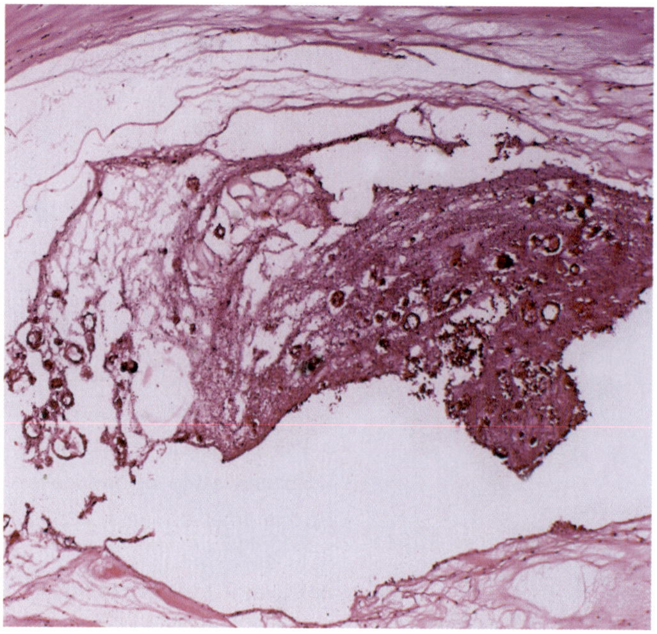

Fig. 7-19. Sagittal section from the intervertebral disc of the lumbar region taken at one year of age, showing notochordal cells and chondrocyte-like cells. The nucleus pulposus is an oval gelatinous mass which occupies the central portion of the disc.

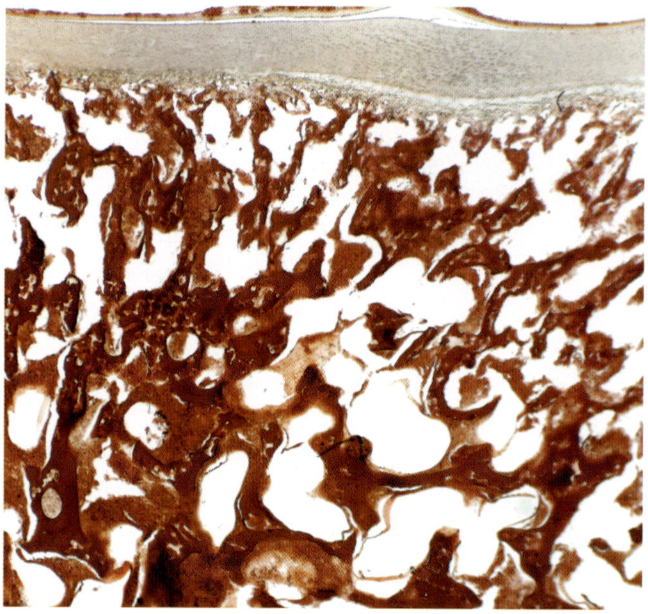

Fig. 7-20. Frontal section of a body of the lumbar vertebra taken at one year of age, showing the endochondral trabeculae in the body. Hematopoietic cells are seen between the trabeculae. Columnar cartilaginous epiphyseal structure is also seen.

References

Jung ST, Nam KI, Kim BY, Yoon JR: The role of cartilage canals in osteogenesis and growth of the vertebrae in the human fetuses. *Korean J Electron Microscopy* 31: 287-305, 2001.

O'Rahilly R, Muller F, Meyer DB: The human vertebral column at the end of the embryonic period proper. *J Anat* 131: 565-575, 1980.

Sensenig EC: The early development of the human vertebral column. *Contrib Embryol Carnegie Inst* 33: 21-41, 1949.

Walmsley R: The development and growth of intervertebral disc. *Edinb Med* 60: 341-364, 1953.

Wilsman NJ, Van Sickle DC: Cartilage canals, their morphology and distribution. *Anat Rec* 173: 79-94, 1972.

Yoon JR, Bae CS, Kim EK: Ultrastructural study on the development of notochordal cells in nucleus pulposus of human fetuses. *Korean J Electron Microscopy* 21: 39-56, 1991.

The Development of the Shoulder Joint

Chapter 08

The development of the shoulder joint is basically similar to that of the knee, hip, and elbow joints. The cartilaginous models of the pectoral girdle and upper limb bones appear slightly before than those of the pelvic girdle and lower limbs. The clavicle initially develops by intramembranous ossification, and it later forms a growth plate.

The chondrification of the humerus at the diaphysis appears in the fetus of the 16 mm embryo (Fig. 8-1), and it extends toward the proximal and distal epiphysis, and in the 25 mm embryo it is completed (Fig. 8-2). The chondrification of the scapula makes its first appearance in the neck, the body, the spine, and acromion process in the 16 mm embryo and reaches completion in the 25 mm embryo. The head of the humerus is, in the 20 to 25 mm embryos, hemispherical and distinct from the diaphysis, and the glenoid is discernible as the concave fossa with the tubercles of many forms. By the 25 mm embryo, the general form of the skeletal elements of the shoulder joint resembles that of the adult. The ossification center of the humerus is present in the 40 mm fetus, and in the 55 mm fetus it extends for nearly one-third of the total length of the humerus. The ossification center of the scapula appears in the 35 to 40 mm fetuses, and the contour of the articular bone is similar to that of the adult. The cartilage canals of the humerus are first seen in the proximal epiphysis in the 55 mm fetus (Fig. 8-8), and in the distal epiphysis in the 60 mm fetus. The endochondral ossification of the humerus is first noted in the 40 mm fetus. Vascularization of the proximal epiphyses begins in the 55 mm fetus, and the resulting cartilage canals increase in size and number during later stages (Figs. 8-10, 8-23, and 8-25). By the 55 mm fetus, the ossification center in the body of the scapula extends into the spine (Fig. 8-9), and by the 90 mm fetus, reaches the base of the acromial process (Fig. 8-14). By the 90 mm fetus, ossification of the shaft of the humerus extends proximally to the level of the teres major muscles (Fig. 8-13). Cartilage canals appear in the head of the scapula in the 100 mm fetus (Fig. 8-15).

The clavicle begins to ossify before any other bone in the body. In the 16 mm embryo, ossification of the clavicle commences with the centers of membranous bone (Fig. 8-2). The clavicle consists mostly of bone in the 170 mm fetus (Fig. 8-15).

The fetal developmental pattern of the shoulder joint is basically similar to the hip joint. In the 13 mm embryo, the homogenus interzone appears (Fig. 8-1), and it is divided into a three-layered interzone in the 25 mm embryo (Fig. 8-3). Its intermediate layer is incorporated into the adjacent chondrogenous layer, while the vascular invasion is present in the 40 mm fetus (Fig. 8-7). The primitive joint cavity is recognized as the primitive form at the interspace of the head of the humerus and the biceps brachii muscle in the 30 mm fetus (Fig. 8-5) and complete in the 35 to 40 mm fetuses (Figs. 8-6 and 8-7). The synovial tissue of the specimens of 90 and 100 mm is more vascular than that of earlier stages and is vascular near the free margin of the glenoid labrum (Fig. 8-16).

The acromioclavicular joint cavity is first seen in the 40 mm fetus without the three-layered interzone (Fig. 8-7). By the 60 and 70 mm fetuses, the acromioclavicular joint is visible (Figs. 8-10 and 8-12). The glenoid labrum appears in the 25 mm embryo as a cellular condensation at the margin of the future glenoid fossa (Fig. 8-3). The labrum becomes very obvious in the 30 mm fetus (Fig. 8-5). By the 55 mm fetus, the labrum is composed of collagenous bundles and cells, and is clearly demarcated from the adjacent hyaline cartilage. In the specimens of 210 and 240 mm, the glenoid labrum is densely fibrous. At the inferior aspect of the joint, the capsule inserts into the labrum and also at its reflection to the humerus, the capsule is quite thick (Figs. 8-12, 8-22, and 8-25).

Development of the extracapsular ligaments, tendons, and bursae can be seen in the 25 mm embryo (Figs. 8-3 and 8-4). Fine collagenous fibers are present in the different ligaments in the 40 mm fetus. All ligaments are more sharply defined in the 60 mm fetus but are still comprised largely of cells (Fig. 8-11). The tendons of the supraspinatus, infraspintus, teres minor, and subscapularis are definite by the 25mm embryo, and they blend with the capsule (Figs. 8-15 and 8-24). The transition of the musculotendinous junction is abrupt in the 90 mm fetus (Fig. 8-13), whereas it is more gradual in the specimens of 110, 130, and 160 mm (Figs. 8-17, 8-19, and 8-20). Blood vessels are present in the tendon of the rotator cuff muscles in the 130 mm fetus (Fig. 8-18). The long tendon of the biceps brachii muscle is present in the 14 mm and 16 mm embryos by the condensation which is continuous with the densely-arranged cells in the anterosuperior part of the interzone. The long bicipital tendon is densely cellular in a 25 mm embryo (Fig. 8-4). A condensation for the tendon of the long head of the triceps brachii muscle is seen at this stage (Fig. 8-3). The subacromial and subscapular bursae are first observed in the 40 mm fetus (Fig. 8-7) and constantly present after the 55 mm fetus. Definite communication between the subscapular bursa and joint cavity is observed first in the 130 mm fetus (Fig. 8-18).

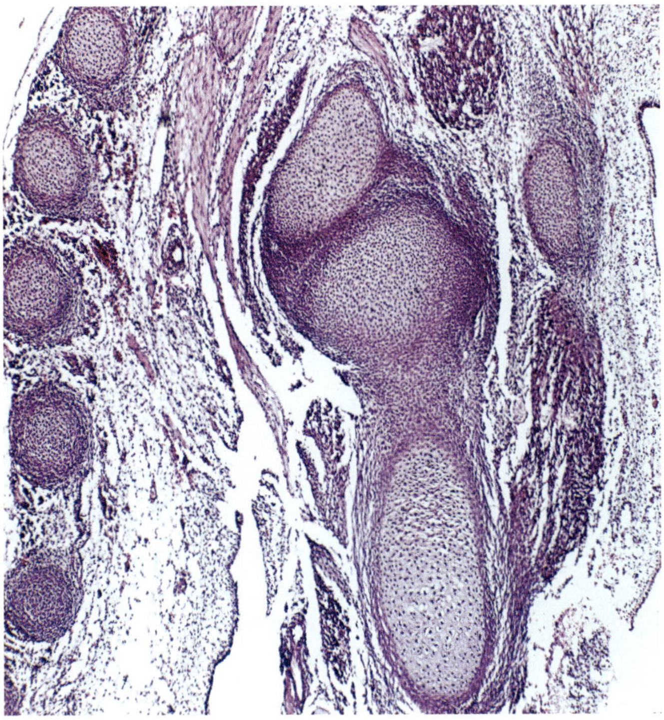

Fig. 8-1. Frontal section of the shoulder from a 13 mm embryo, illustrating the early interzone between the humeral head and glenoid. The cartilaginous models of the glenoid and humeral head are separated by a homogenous interzone. Condensation of the glenoid labrum is evident, and the tendon of the biceps brachii adjacent to humerus is barely visible. The acromion also begins to chondrify.

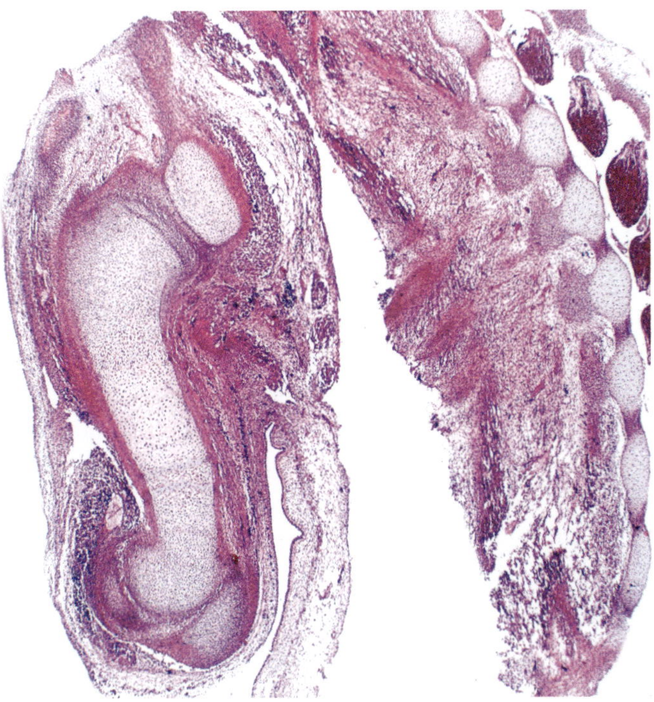

Fig. 8-2. Frontal section of shoulder from a 16 mm embryo to show chondrification of the humerus. The clavicle is ossifying. The deltoid and triceps brachii can be seen. At the right border, the cartilaginous ribs are clearly visible.

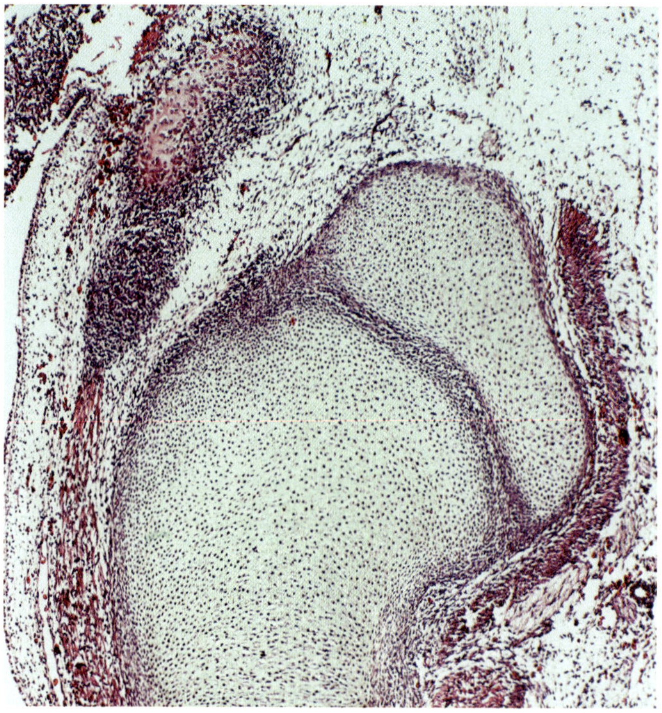

Fig. 8-3. Frontal section of the shoulder in the 25 mm embryo to show the three-layered interzone. The deltoid and long head of the triceps brachii can be seen. Condensation for the glenoid labrum is evident. The membranous bone formation of the clavicle is defined.

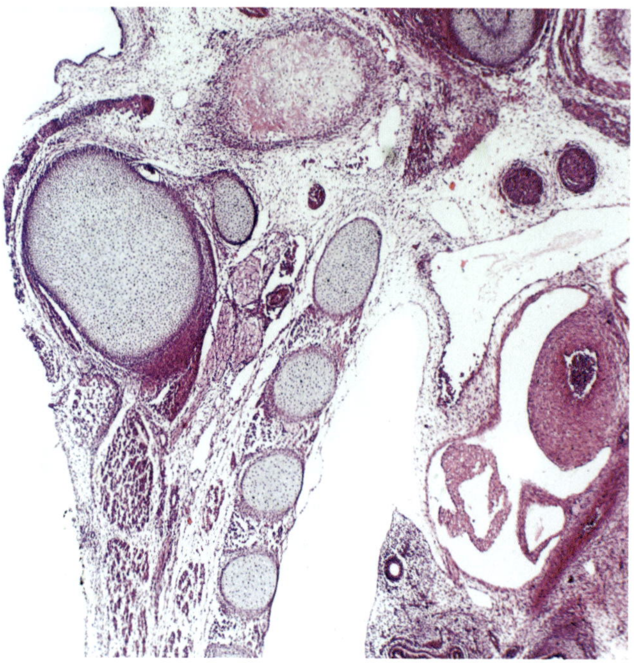

Fig. 8-4. Frontal section through the shoulder joint in the 25 mm embryo to show the head of the humerus. The long head of the biceps brachii in the intertubercular groove is defined. The deltoid and axillary sheath are seen.

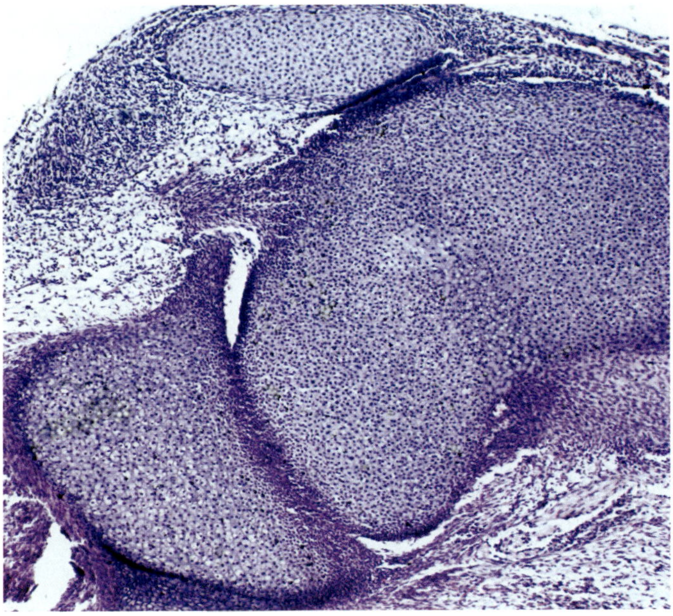

Fig. 8-5. Frontal section of the shoulder from a 30 mm fetus to show cavitation at the periphery of the interzone. Note the well-defined glenoid labrum.

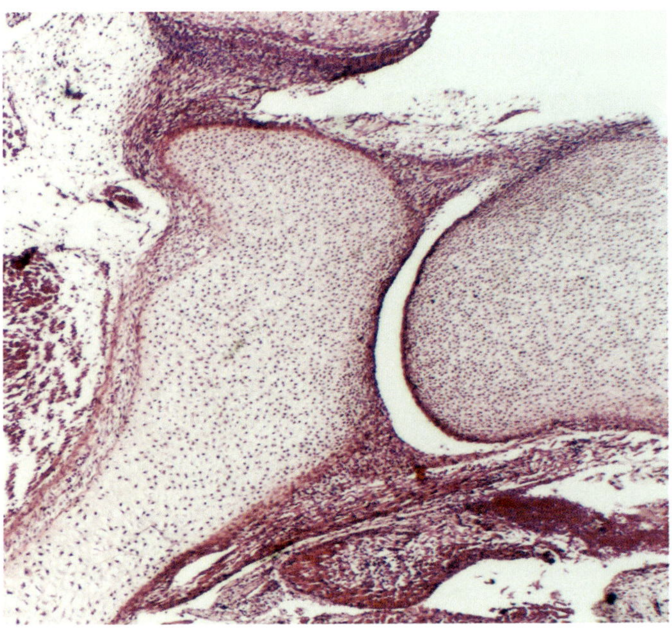

Fig. 8-6. Frontal section of the shoulder joint in the 35 mm fetus, showing the well-formed glenohumeral joint. The cavity is well developed. The glenoid labrum is more marked on the superior margin.

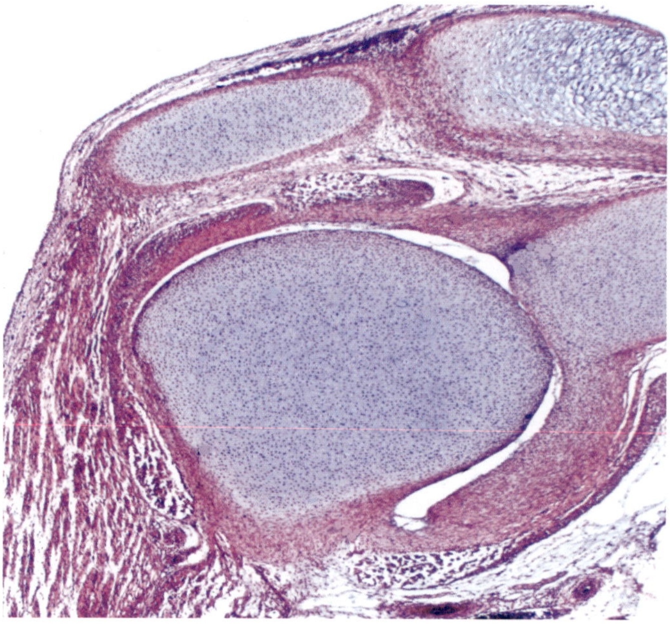

Fig. 8-7. Frontal section of the shoulder joint from a 40 mm fetus to show the cavity around the head of the humerus. Note the well-defined glenoid labrum and the capsule. The supraspinatus is closely adherent to the joint capsule. The subacromial bursa starts to form. A cavity of the acromioclavicular joint is not seen.

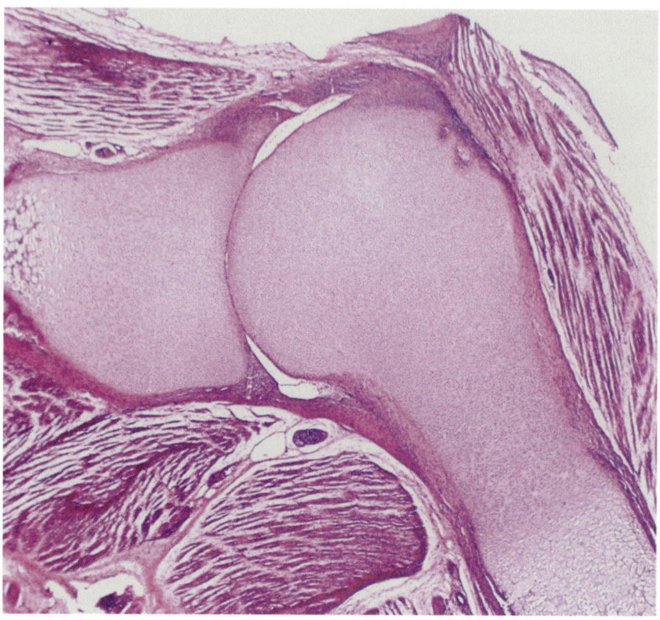

Fig. 8-8. Frontal section of the shoulder joint in a 55 mm fetus to show the glenoid cavity. The inferior capsule is thick, irregular, and richly cellular. The fusion of the tendon of the supraspinatus and joint capsule is clearly visible. Cartilage canals appear in the proximal humeral epiphysis.

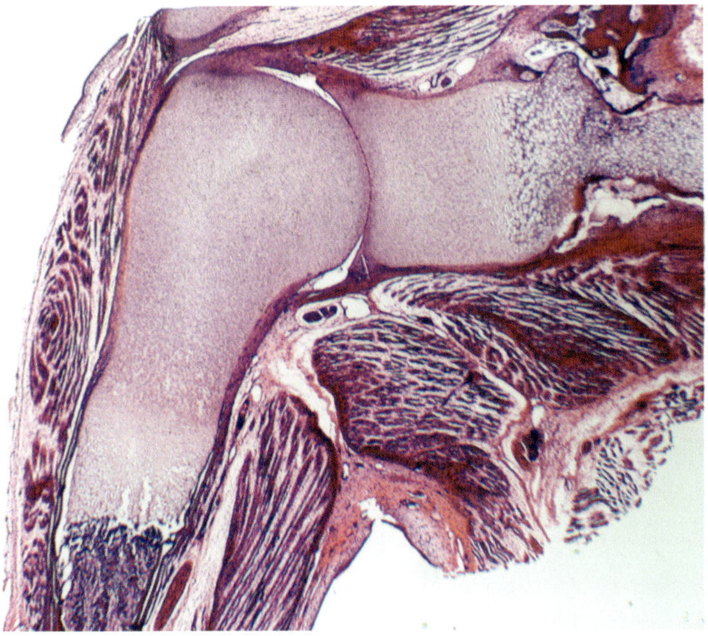

Fig. 8-9. Frontal section through the shoulder joint in a 55 mm fetus to show the extent of the endochondral ossification of the scapula and the humerus. The suprascapular nerve and artery can be seen.

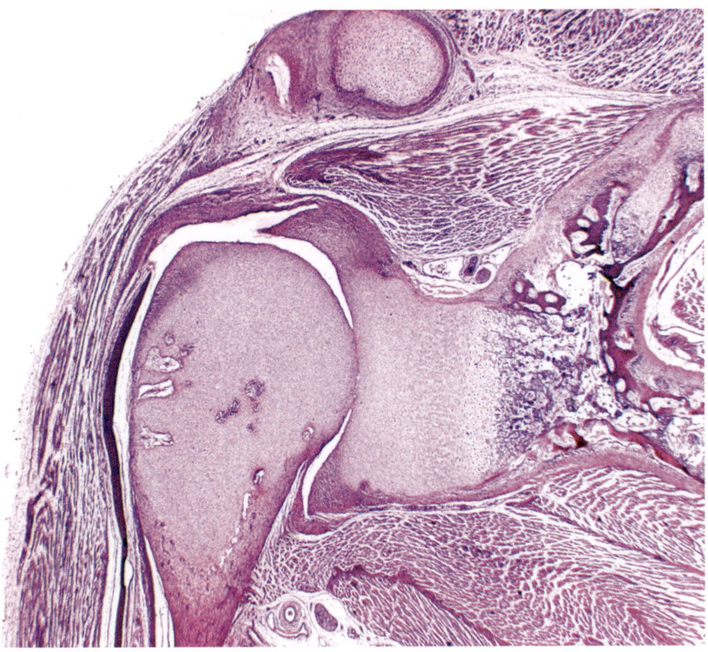

Fig. 8-10. Frontal section of the shoulder joint from a 60 mm fetus to show cartilage canals in the proximal humeral epiphysis. The endochondral ossification of the scapula is spreading from the body toward the glenoid cavity. The tendon of the biceps brachii lay free in the joint cavity. The cavity in acromioclavicular joint appears.

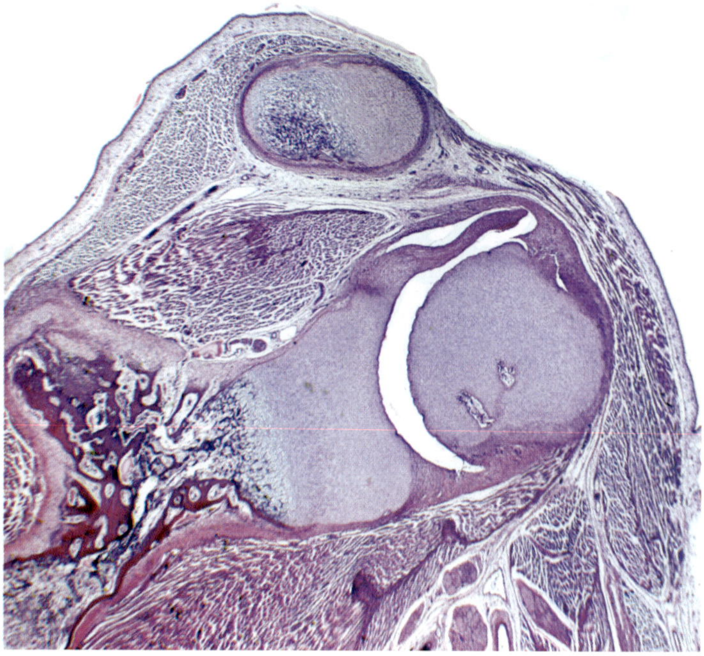

Fig. 8-11. Frontal section through the shoulder joint from a 60 mm fetus to show the glenoid cavity. The inferior joint capsule is thick. The section includes the origin of the long head of the biceps brachii.

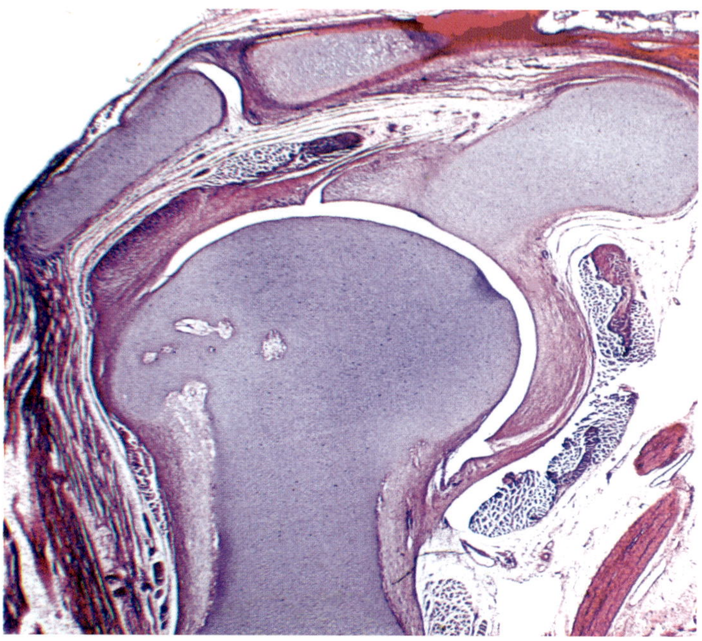

Fig. 8-12. Frontal section of the shoulder joint in a 70 mm fetus to show a vascular channel communicating between epiphysis and diaphysis. The acromioclavicular joint cavity is completed. The inferior joint recess is well-formed. The subacromial bursa is seen.

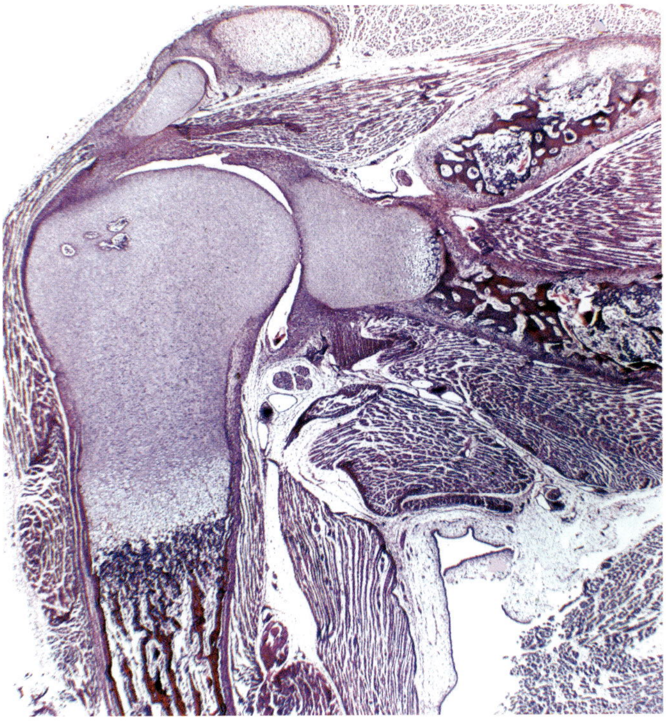

Fig. 8-13. Frontal section of the shoulder joint from a 90 mm fetus to show the acromioclavicular and glenohumeral joints. The supraspinatus tendon is seen blending with the capsule. Vascular invasion of the head of the humerus is shown. The suprascapular nerve and artery can be seen in the scapular notch. The axillary sheath is also observed. The inferior synovial recess is shown.

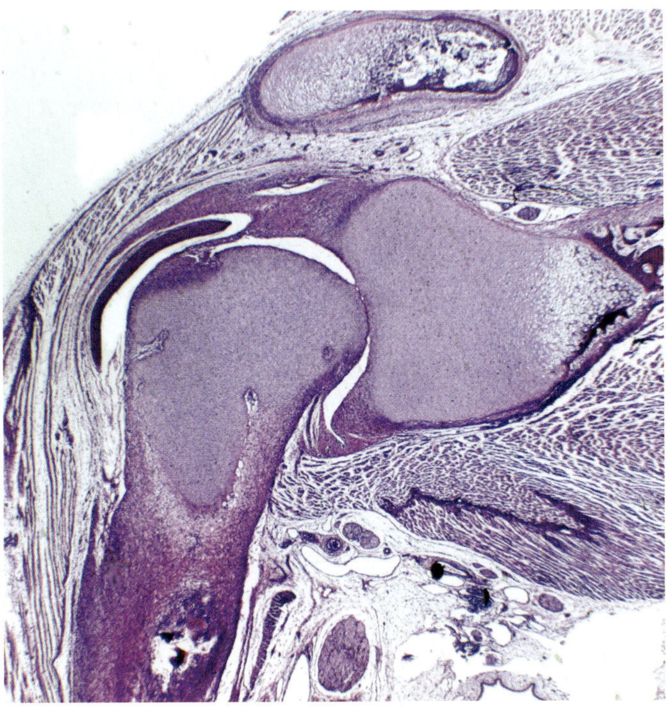

Fig. 8-14. Frontal section of the shoulder joint from a 90 mm fetus to show the superior and inferior glenoid labra. The tendon of the biceps brachii lay free in the joint cavity. The axillary sheath is seen in the axilla. The supurascapular nerve and artery can be seen in the scapular notch. Note the advancing endochondral ossification of the scapula.

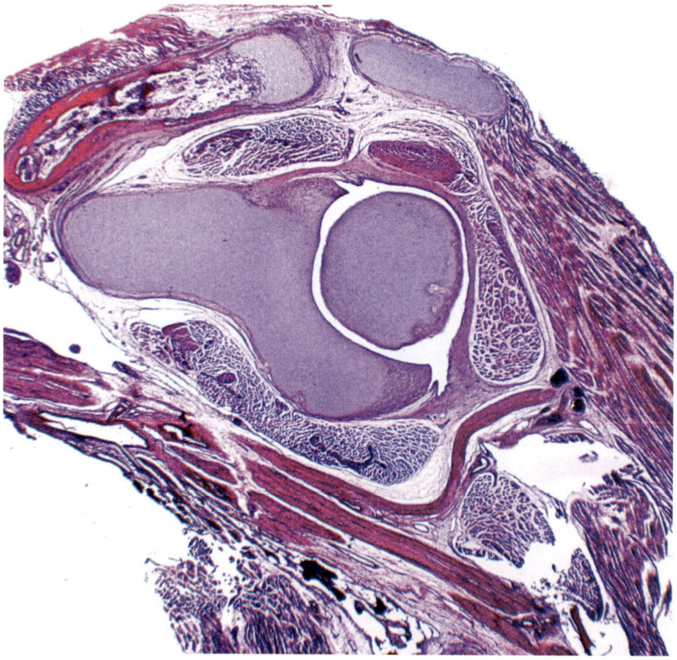

Fig. 8-15. Transverse section through the shoulder joint in a 100 mm fetus to show cartilage canals in the head of scapula and humerus. The tendons of the supraspinatus, infraspinatus, teres minor, and subscapularis blend with the capsule. The endochondral ossification of the clavicle is spreading from the center of the shaft toward both ends. The brachial plexus is observed.

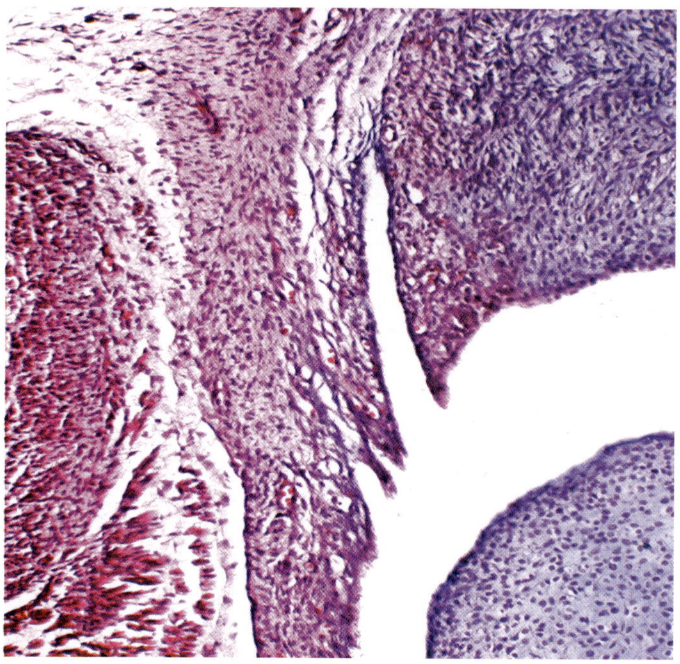

Fig. 8-16. Transverse section through the shoulder joint from a 100 mm fetus to show the glenoid labrum. Cellular and vascular synovial tissue near the glenoid labrum is seen.

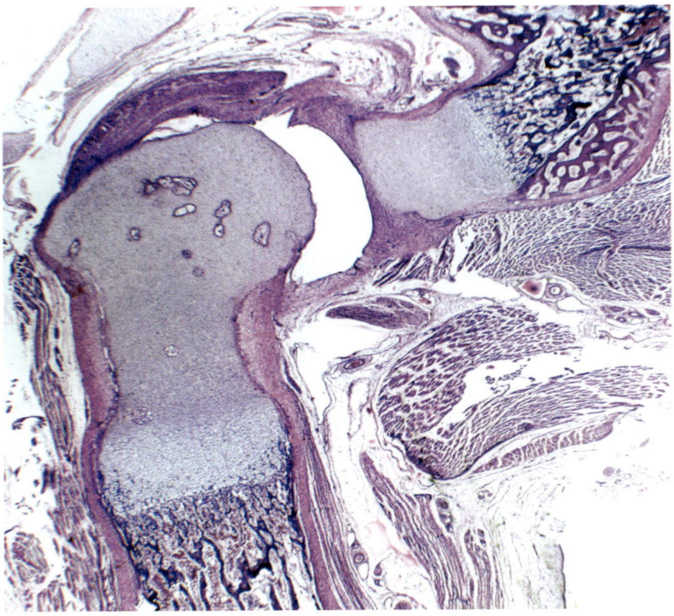

Fig. 8-17. Frontal section of the shoulder joint from a 110 mm fetus, showing the glenoid labra. The tendinous portion of the supuraspnatus blends with the capsule. Cartilage canals in the head of the humerus are seen.

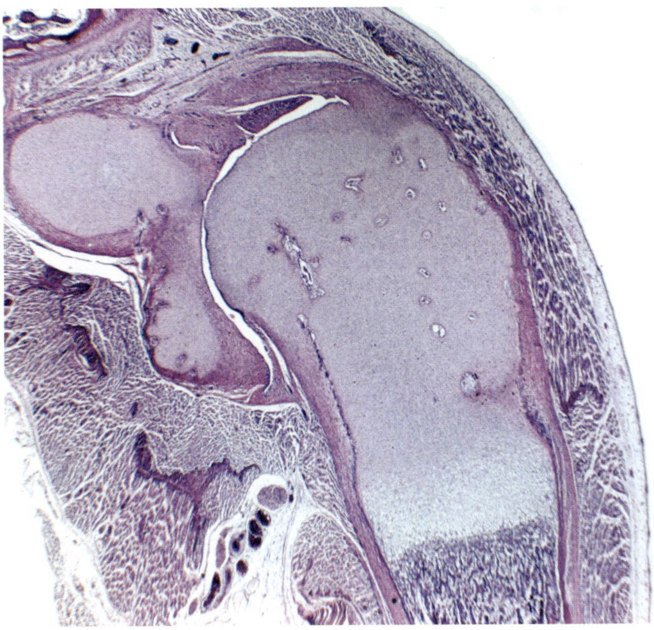

Fig. 8-18. Frontal section of the shoulder from a 130 mm fetus to show communication of subscapular bursa and joint cavity. The tendon of the supuraspinatus and its insertion on the greater tubercle of the humerus are well identified. The long head of the biceps brachii is covered by the capsule.

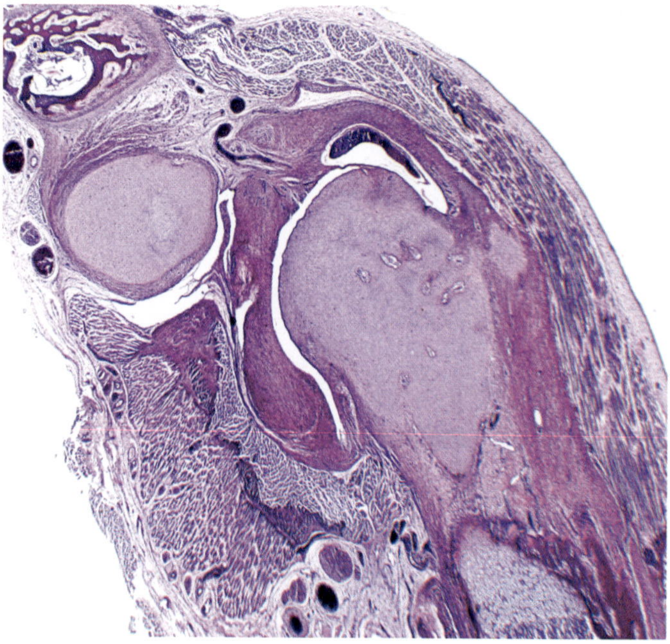

Fig. 8-19. Frontal section through the shoulder joint in a 130 mm fetus to show the redundant inferior capsule. The tendon of biceps brachii and the superior joint capsule are clearly visible.

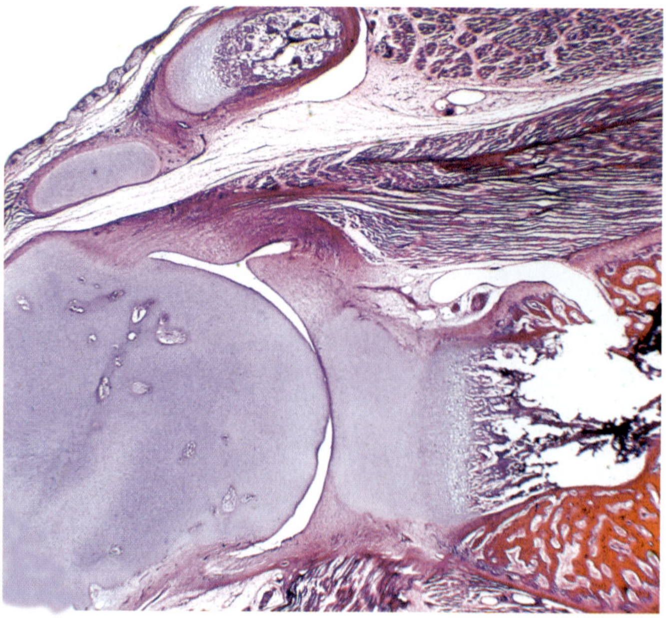

Fig. 8-20. Frontal section through the part of the shoulder joint from a 160 mm fetus, illustrating the joint capsule and labrum. The supraspinatus tendon is closely adherent to the joint capsule. The cartilaginous extremity of the clavicle and subacromial bursa are seen.

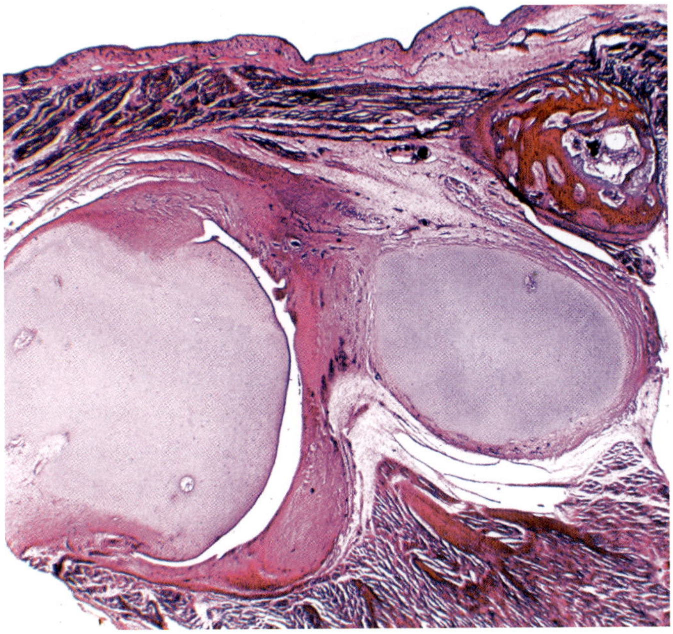

Fig. 8-21. Frontal section through the shoulder joint from a 160 mm fetus to show the joint capsule. The section includes the tendon of the supraspinatus and its insertion on the greater tubercle of the humerus. The superior glenohumeral ligament is seen.

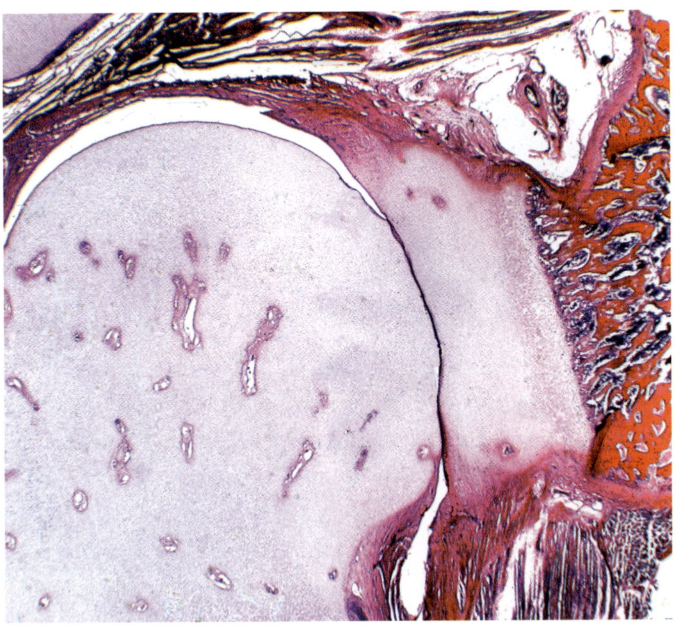

Fig. 8-22. Frontal section through the part of the shoulder joint from a 210 mm fetus to show increased ossification and vascularization at the scapula. Cartilage canals are seen in the humeral head and the neck of the scapula. Note the inferior joint recess.

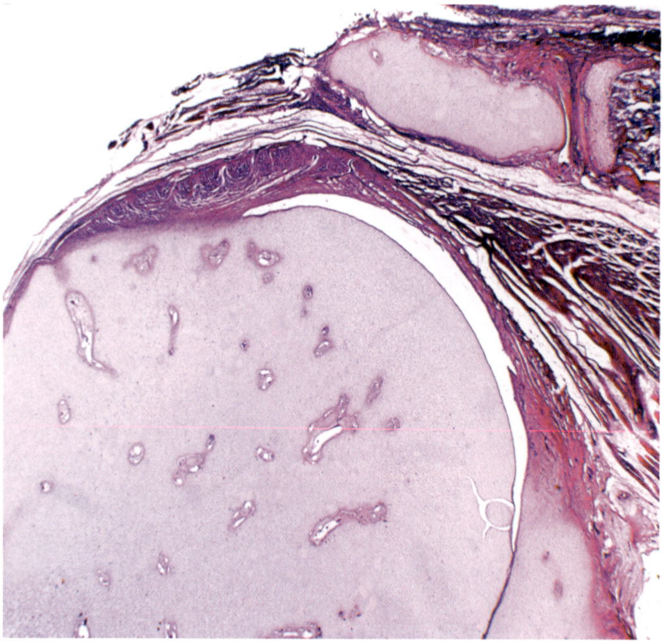

Fig. 8-23. Frontal section through the shoulder and acromioclavicular joints from a 210 mm fetus to show the superior capsule and glenoidal labrum. The tendons of the supraspinatus and infraspinatus blend with the capsule. Cartilage canals in the humeral head and acromion are seen.

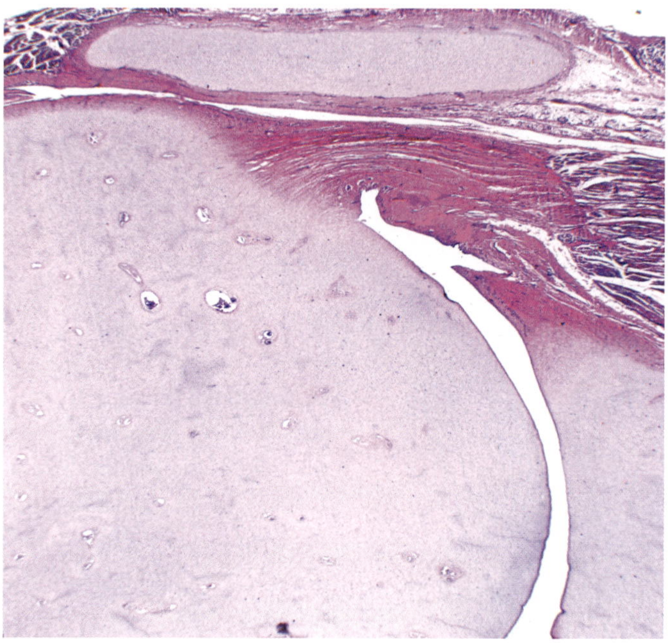

Fig. 8-24. Frontal section through the shoulder joint in a 230 mm fetus to show the glenoidal labrum. The tendon of the supraspinatus is closely adherent to the capsule. The subacromial bursa is clearly visible.

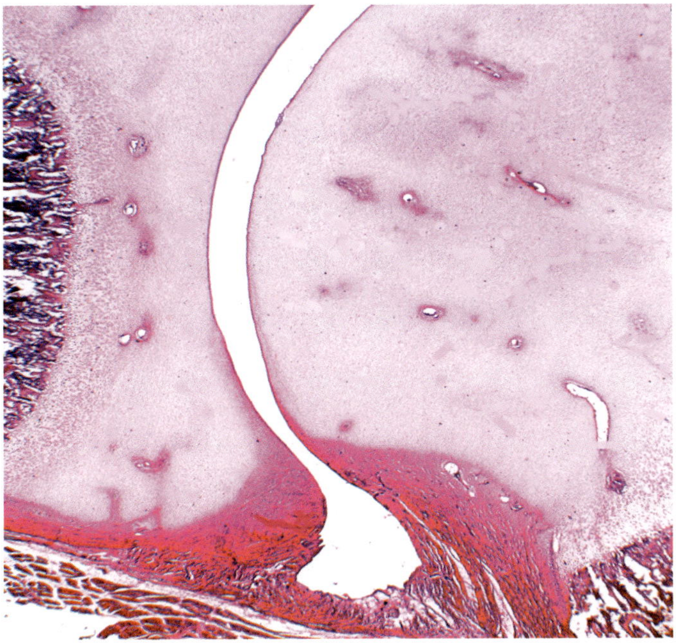

Fig. 8-25. Frontal section through the part of the shoulder joint from a 240 mm fetus, illustrating particularly the thick capsule inferiorly. Cartilage canals are longer and numerous in the head of the humerus and the neck of the scapula.

References

Gardner E, Gray DJ: Prenatal development of the human shoulder and acromioclavicualar joints. *Am J Anat* 92: 219-276, 1953.

Gray DJ, Gardner E: The prenatal development of the human elbow joint. *Am J Anat* 88: 429-470, 1951.

Haines RW: The development of joints. *J Anat* 81: 33-55, 1947.

Song SJ: The prenatal development of the shoulder joint in Korean fetus. *Chonnam Medical J* 8: 645-660, 1971.

The Development of the Elbow Joint

Chapter 09

The elbow joint consists mainly of condensed blastemal tissue in the 12 mm embryo (Fig. 9-1). By the 16 mm embryo, the distal end of the humerus, the blastemal condensation, is enlarged to form the condyles. At this stage, the olecranon process can be distinguished and cartilage cells in the radius and ulna begin to enlarge (Fig. 9-2). The head and neck of the radius are clearly defined and the radial notch is evident in the 35 mm fetus (Fig. 9-5). The form of the skeletal elements at this stage corresponds to that of the adult elbow joint. The primary ossification center of the radius is evident at this stage. By the 50 mm fetus, ossification of the radius has progressed proximally almost to the level of the radial tuberosity and has reached approximately the same level in the ulna. Ossification nearly extends the radial neck by the 150 mm fetus. In the ulna, it extends almost to the coronoid process (Fig. 9-18). By the 200 mm fetus, the radius is ossified to a level proximal to the neck, and in the humerus it extends almost to its condyles (Fig. 9-20).

The initial phases of vascularization of the humeral epiphyses are recognized in the 90 mm fetus. The early appearance of cartilage canals of the humerus is first seen in the distal epiphysis in the 100 mm fetus (Fig. 9-14). The cartilage canals appear in the olecranon process by the 100 mm fetus, and in the head of the radius by the 130 mm fetus (Fig. 9-16). During the growth of the epiphyses, the cartilage canals are numerous and occasionally communicate with channels in the diaphyses (Figs. 9-17 and 9-19). The cartilage canals are observed to contain a number of thin-walled blood vessels and loose connective tissue. The vessels originate from the perichondral vascular network and some of them communicate with those in the diaphysis.

The homogenous interzone and three-layered interzone in the elbow joint are present in the 16 mm and 24 mm embryos (Figs. 9-2 and 9-3). Recognition of the radiohumeral and ulnohumeral cavities is possible in the 30 to 35 mm fetuses (Figs. 9-4 and 9-5), while the proximal radioulnar cavity is observed for the first time in the 50 mm fetus (Fig. 9-7). Synovial folds, appearing in the 40 mm fetus, are infiltrated first by numerous blood vessels (Fig. 9-6). The synovial folds are richly vascularized (Figs. 9-10, 9-12, and 9-13). Collagenous fibers in synovial tissue in the 60 mm fetus are small, irregularly arranged, and deep to the fibrous capsule (Fig. 9-8). Larger numbers of collagenous fibers are present in the synovial tissue in the 150 mm fetus (Fig. 9-18). Adipose tissue is present for the first time at this stage, and elastic fibers can be seen in the specimen at term (Fig. 9-21).

The capsule and tendon are noted as cellular condensation around most of the joint in the 20 mm embryo. Collagenous fibers are found in those condensations in the 30 mm fetus, and their presence clearly defines the annular and collateral ligaments. The annular ligament is seen over the radial head, and it continues into the capsule (Fig. 9-6). The radial and ulnar collateral ligaments are densely collagenous by the 70 mm fetus, and the annular ligament shows clearly the circular arrangement of the majority of its fibers. The annular ligament is seen over the radial head and it continues into the capsule throughout the fetal life (Figs. 9-9, 9-11, 9-15, and 9-20).

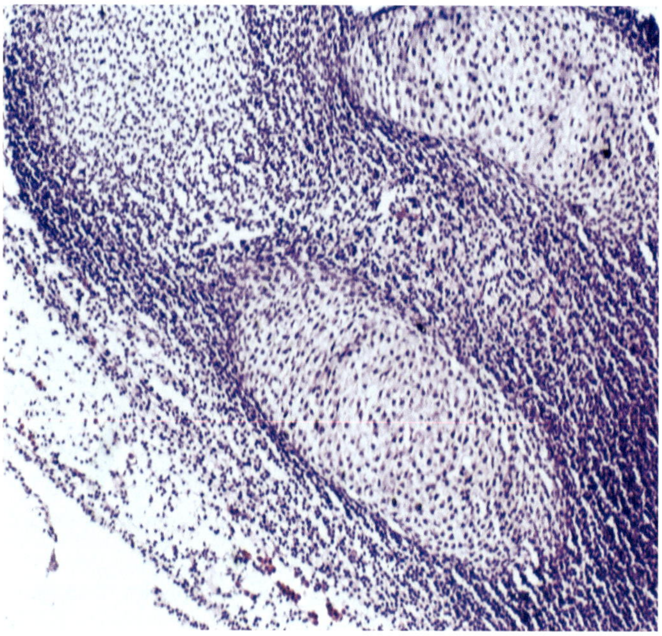

Fig. 9-1. Sagittal section through the elbow region of a 14 mm embryo, showing cellular condensation between humerus and ulna. A thick interzone separates the two chondrifications and gives the first indication of the joint formation.

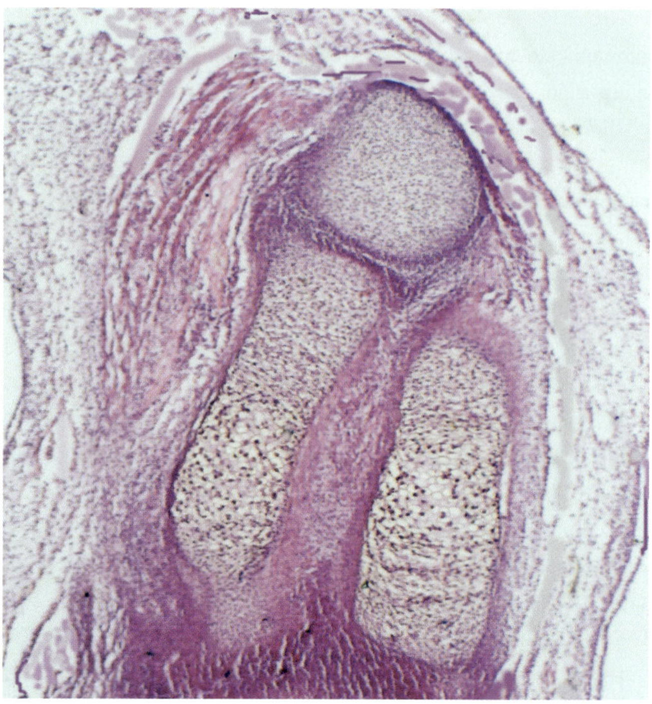

Fig. 9-2. Sagittal section through the elbow joint from a 17 mm embryo, showing the interzone between the humerus and radius. The trochlear region of the humerus is separated from the ulna by a thick interzone.

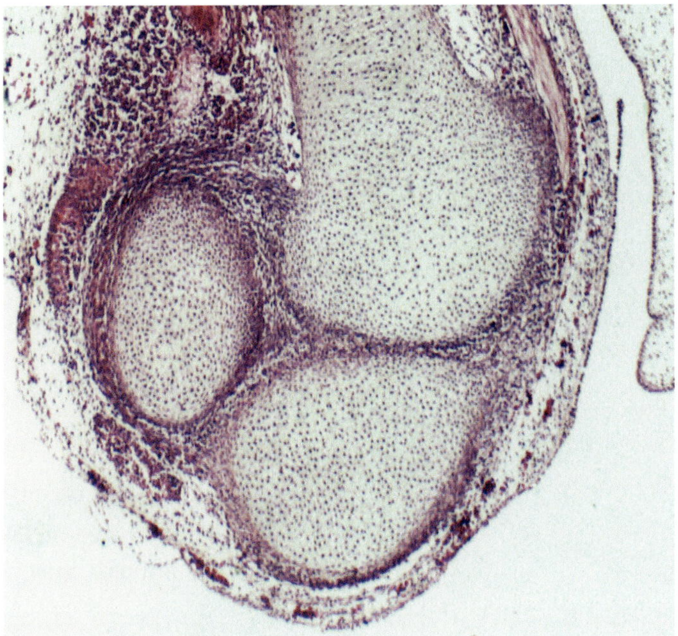

Fig. 9-3. Sagittal section through humerus, radius, and ulna from a 24 mm embryo, showing the three-layered arrangement of the humeroradial and humeroulnar interzones. The median and ulnar nerves are seen.

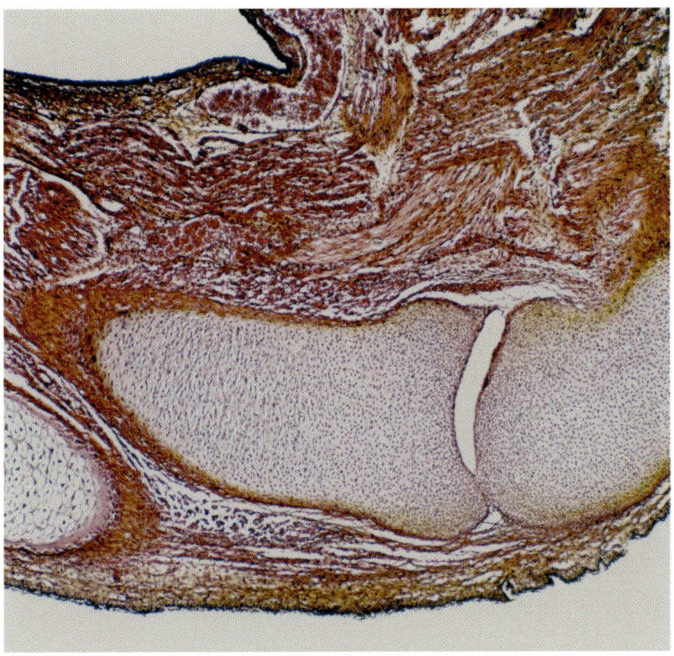

Fig. 9-4. Sagittal section through the distal humerus, radius and a part of ulna from a 30 mm embryo to show the cavity of the humeroradial joint. A condensation for the capsule is most evident anteriorly in the region of annular ligament.

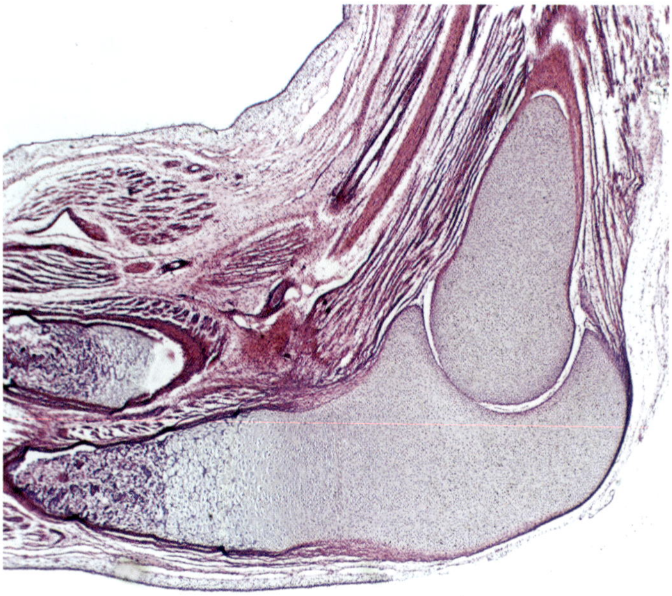

Fig. 9-5. Sagittal section through the humerus, radius, and ulna from a 35 mm fetus to show the humeroulnar joint. The formation of the cavity in the humeroulnar interzone is evident. The brachialis and triceps brachii muscles are seen. The median nerve and brachial artery are also seen.

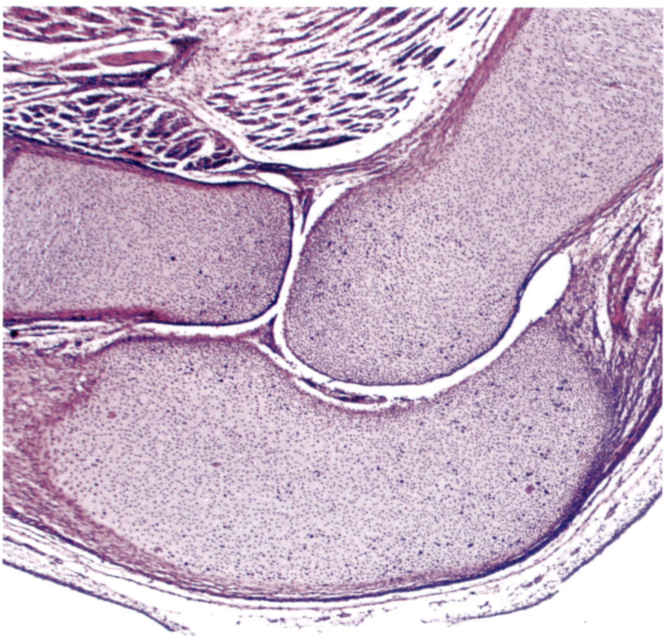

Fig. 9-6. Sagittal section through humerus, radius, and part of ulna from a 40 mm fetus to show the humeroradial, humeroulnar, and proximal radioulnar joints. A condensation for the capsule is present anteriorly in region of annular ligament. A small, triangular fold of well-vascularized loose tissue extends from the annular ligament, and a similar fold extends from the lateral side of the olecranon.

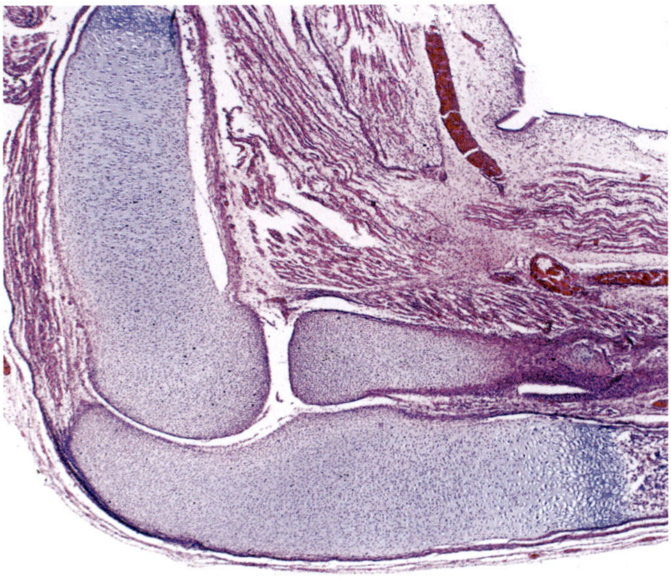

Fig. 9-7. Sagittal section through humerus, radius, and ulna from a 50 mm fetus to show the humeroradial, humeroulnar, and proximal radioulnar joints. A capsule is present only anteriorly. The brachial artery is seen. Note that the radial head is larger than the neck.

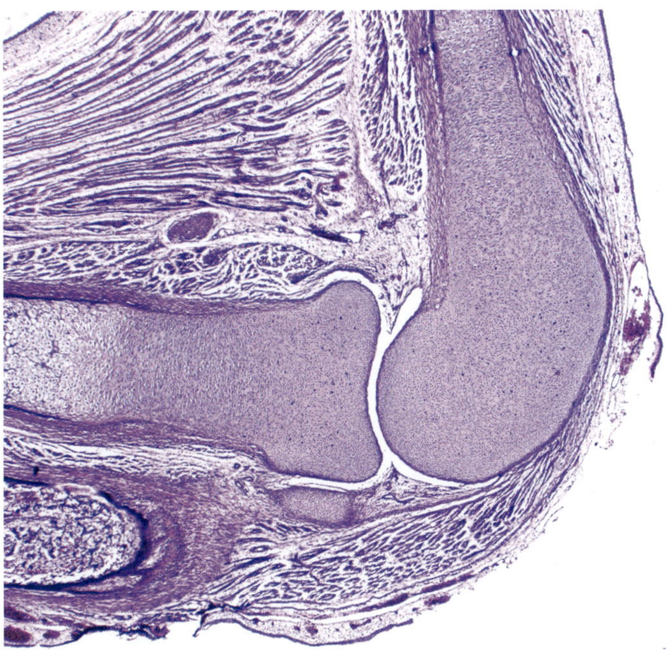

Fig. 9-8. Sagittal section through humerus, radius, and part of ulna from a 60 mm fetus to show the elbow joint. The shape of the radial head resembles its adult form. The annular ligament is seen. The loose cellular fold projects into the joint cavity.

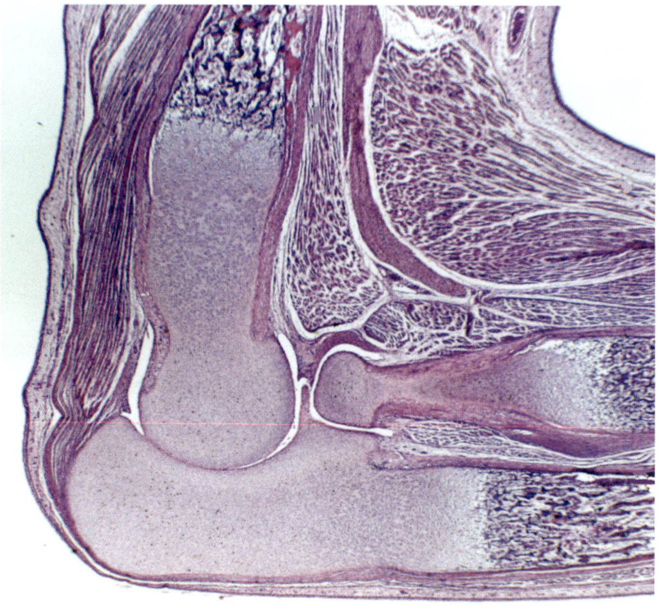

Fig. 9-9. Sagittal section through the elbow joint from a 70 mm fetus to show the humeroulnar and proximal radioulnar joints. The olecranon and coronoid processes start to develop. The median nerve is clearly visible. The lateral fold and annular ligament are also seen. The tendon of the triceps brachii is inserted into the perichondrium of the olecranon.

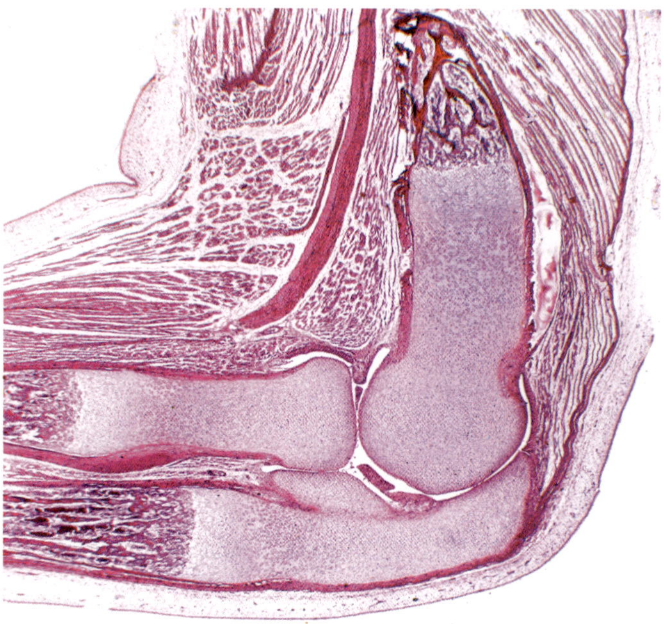

Fig. 9-10. Sagittal section through the elbow joint from a 90 mm fetus to show the humeroulnar, humeroradial, and proximal radioulnar joints. The annular ligament is thick. A portion of the lateral fold projects into the joint cavity and a large fold lies just superior to the olecranon. The median nerve is clearly visible.

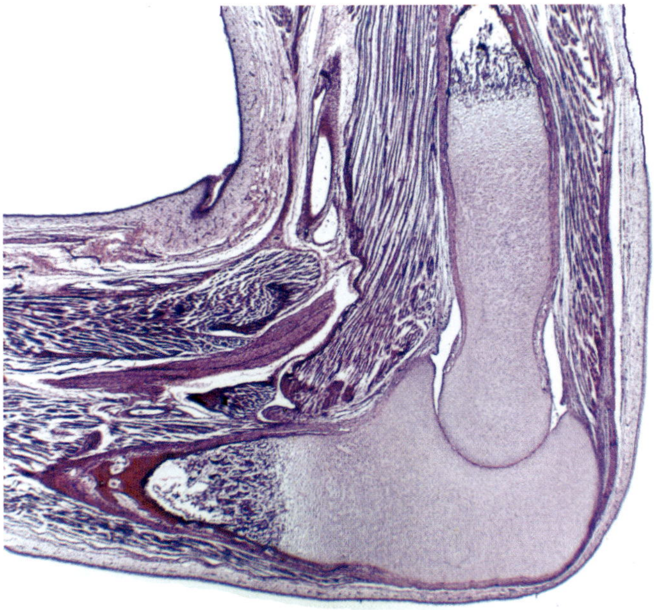

Fig. 9-11. Sagittal section through the humerus, radius, and ulna from a 90 mm fetus to show elbow joint. The olecranon and coronoid fossae are clearly visible. The brachial artery and median nerve are seen. The tendinous insertions of the brachialis and triceps brachii are also seen.

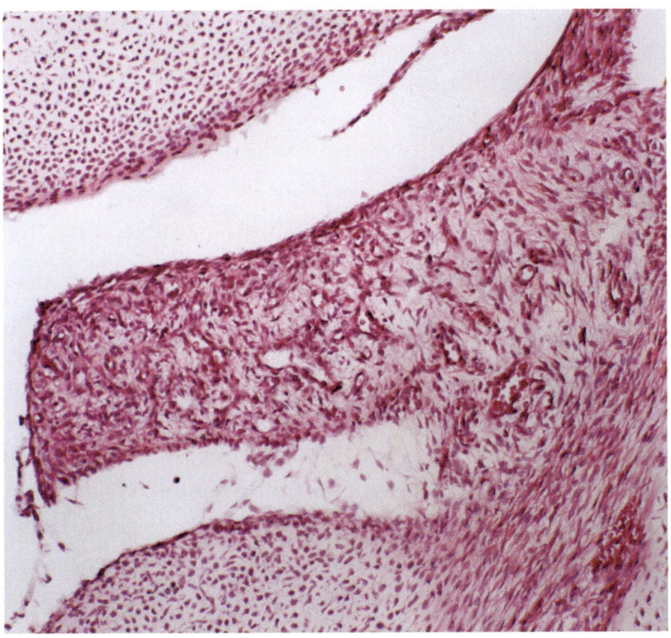

Fig. 9-12. Sagittal section through the elbow joint in a 90 mm fetus to show the synovial fold. A villus extends from the synovial lining into the proximal radioulnar joint. The loose connective tissue comprising the subintima contains several blood vessels.

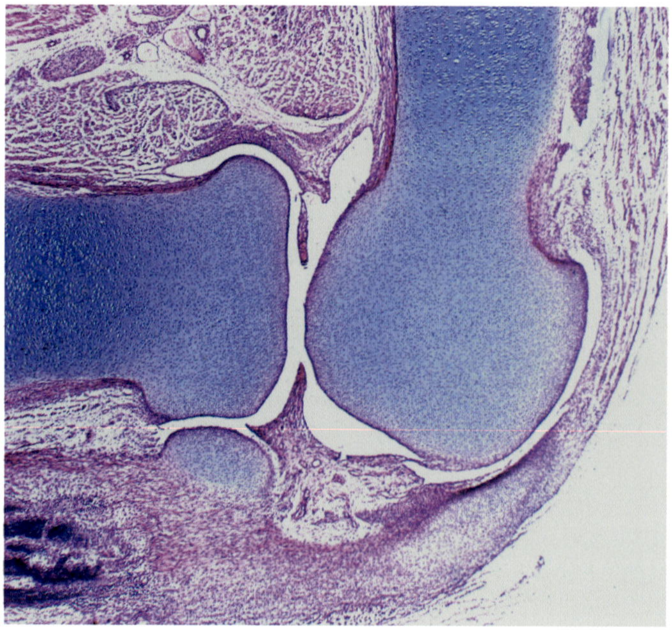

Fig. 9-13. Sagittal section through the humerus, radius and ulna from a 100 mm fetus to show the elbow joint. The annular ligament is thick. A loose vascular fold projects into cavity.

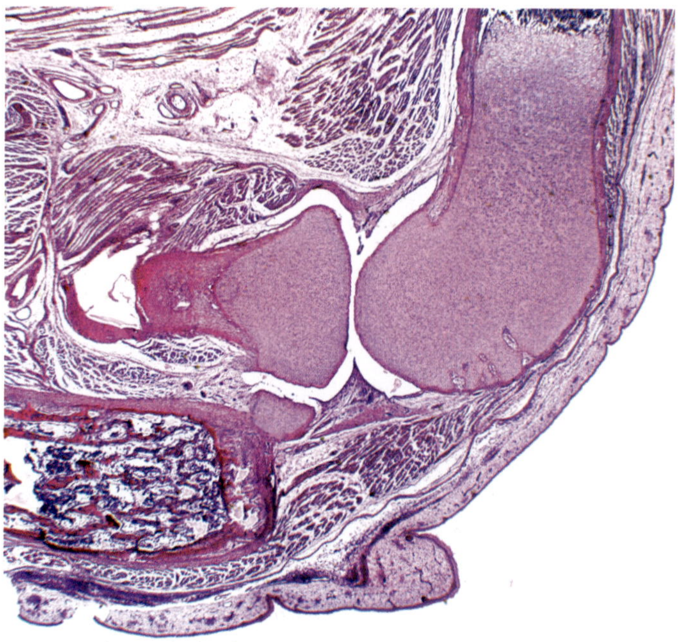

Fig. 9-14. Sagittal section through the elbow joint in a 100 mm fetus to show cartilage canals in the distal epiphysis of the humerus. The lateral fold projects into the joint cavity and a small fold lies in the proximal radioulnar joint cavity.

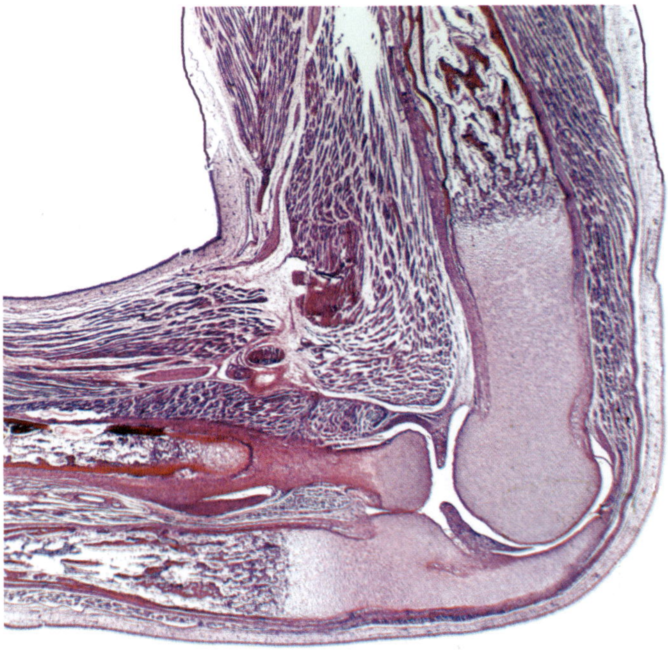

Fig. 9-15. Sagittal section through the humerus, ulna, and radius from a 100 mm fetus to show the elbow joint. The annular ligament is dense and continues into the anterior capsule. A large fold extends into the cavity above the annular ligament. Vascular invasion of the humeral epiphysis starts on its medial and lateral humeral epicondyles.

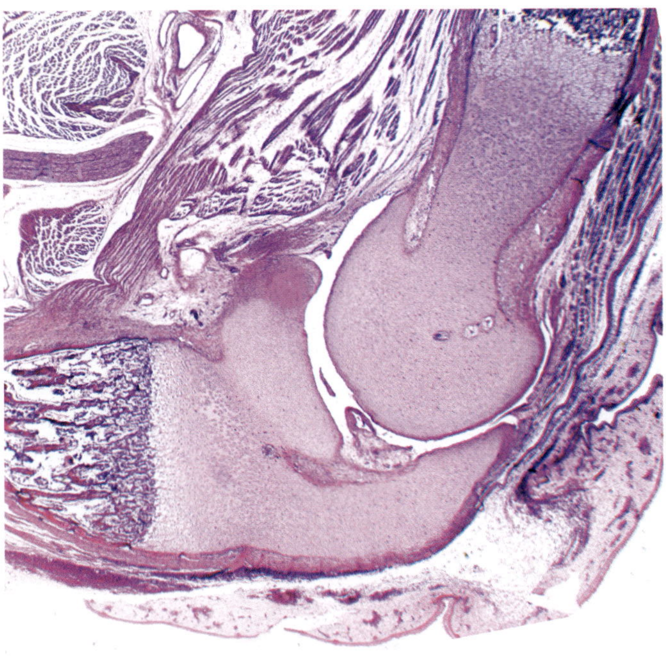

Fig. 9-16. Sagittal section through the elbow joint in a 130 mm fetus to show the vascularization of epiphysis. The cartilage canals in the distal epiphysis of the humerus and proximal epiphysis of the ulna are seen. Note the vascular invasion of the humeral epiphysis from perichondrium. The median nerve lies just anterior to the tendon of the brachialis muscle.

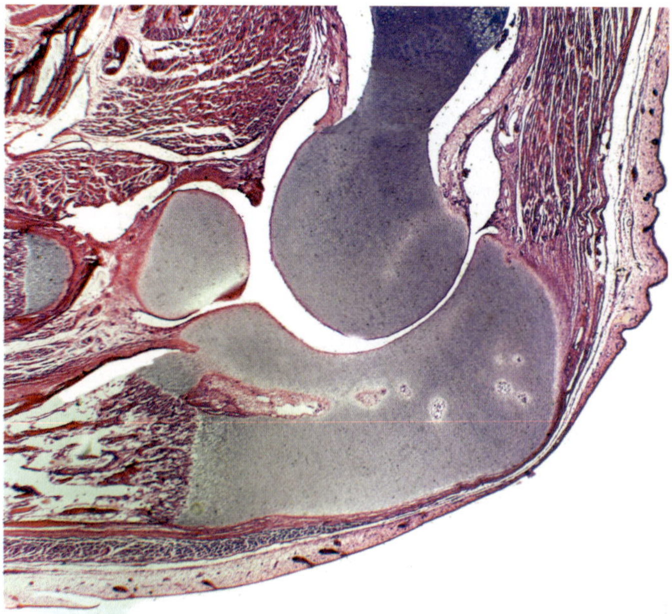

Fig. 9-17. Sagittal section through the humerus, ulna, and part of radius from a 150 mm fetus to show cartilage canals in the olecranon. Note the cartilage canals communicating with vessels in the zone of endochondral ossification of the metaphysis. A portion of the lateral fold projects into the joint cavity and a small fold lies superior to the olecranon process.

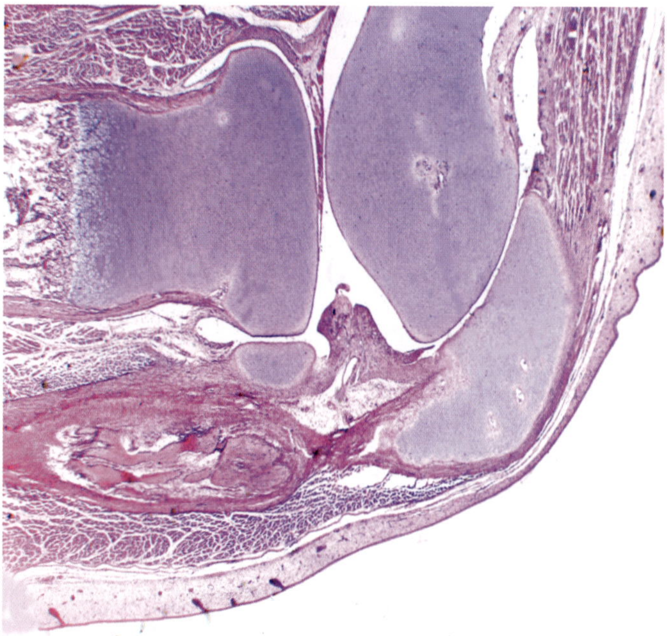

Fig. 9-18. Sagittal section through the humerus, radius, and part of ulna in a 150 mm fetus to show cartilage canals in all three epiphyses. Ossification of the radius extends a level distal to the neck. The synovial folds extend into the cavity above the annular ligament. The capsule lining the inferior part of the proximal radioulnar joint is very thin.

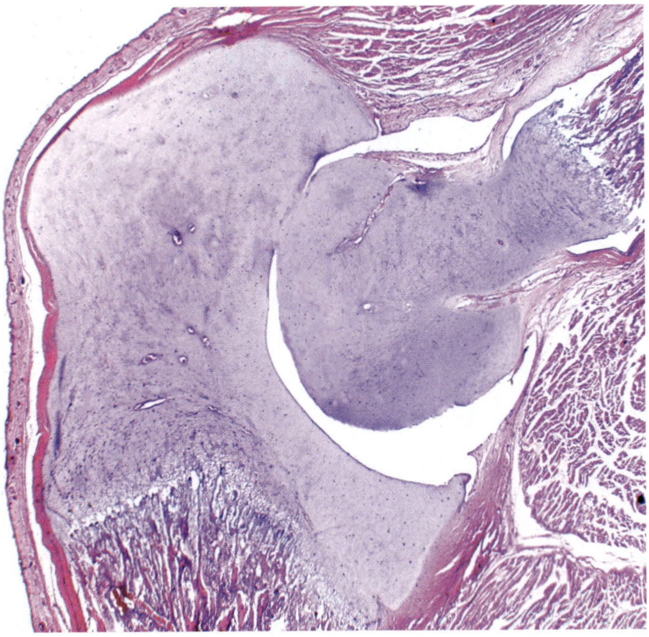

Fig. 9-19. Sagittal section through the humerus and ulna from a 180 mm fetus to show cartilage canals in the condyle of the humerus and olecranon. Ossification in the ulna extends half the distance between the coronoid process and the superior limit of the olecranon. Cartilage canals penetrate the anterior and posterior aspects of the distal extremity of the humerus.

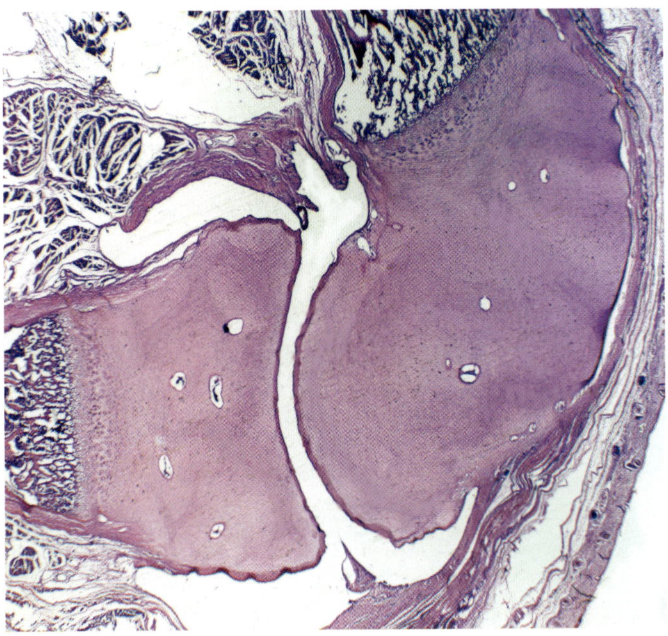

Fig. 9-20. Sagittal section through the elbow joint in the 200 mm fetus to show cartilage canals in the radius and humerus. Ossification of the radius extends a level proximal to the neck, and in the humerus it extends distally to the condyles. Synovial folds extend into the cavity above the annular ligament.

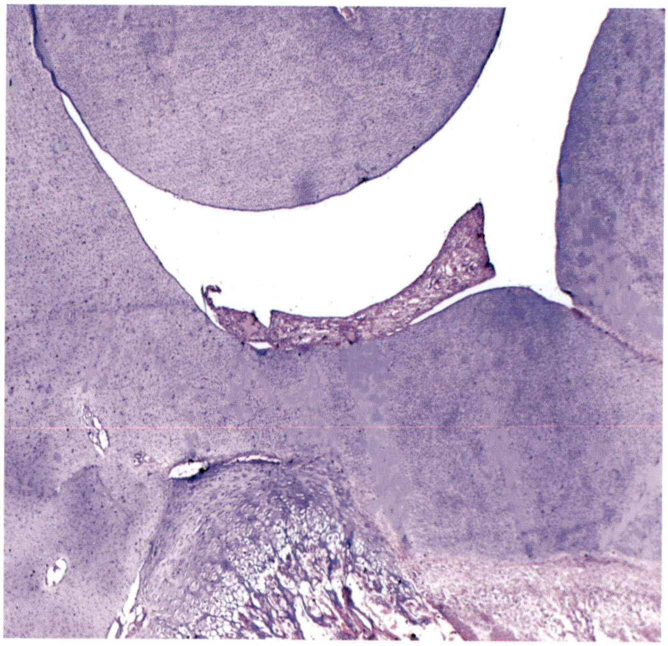

Fig. 9-21. Sagittal section through the humerus, radius, and ulna from a 230 mm fetus to show the humeroulnar, humeroradial, and proximal radioulnar joints. Ossification in the ulna extends to the olecranon. The synovial foid consists of collagenous fibers containing lobules of fat and many blood vessels.

References

Gray DJ, Gardner E: Prenatal development of the human elbow joint. *Am J Anat* 88: 429-470, 1951.

Lee BC: The prenatal development of the elbow joint in Korean fetuses. *Chonnam Medical J* 9: 131-144, 1972.

Martin BF: The annular ligament of the superior radioulnar joint. *J Anat* 92: 473-482, 1958.

The Development of the Wrist and Hand

Chapter 10

In the 10 mm embryo, the carpal region is represented by a mass of condensed blastema. At the wrist, this is continuous proximally with the radius and ulna, and distally with the metacarpals, and in this blastema the elements of the carpus appear as centers of more condensed tissue (Fig. 10-1). The digit begins to chondrify in proximodistal sequence. The anlage of the wrist and hand appears in the 14 mm embryo (Fig. 10-2), and chondrification is complete in the 20 mm embryo (Fig. 10-3). Also at this stage, the elements of the carpus chondrify starting with the capitate and hamate. The lunate and pisiform are the last to chondrify. By the 30 mm fetus, formation of the os centrale between the scaphoid and capitate is established (Fig. 10-4). At the end of embyonic period general form of the skeletal elements in the wrist and hand resemble that of adult.

A primary bone collar and hypertrophied cartilage cells of the metacarpals are first noted in the 35 mm fetus (Fig. 10-7). The first metacarpal bone is the latest of the metacarpals to show evidence of ossification. The endochondral ossification of metacarpals is first noted in the 50 mm fetus (Fig. 10-11). As endochondral ossification proceeds proximally and distally, periosteal bone formation also proceeds longitudinally until about the 220 mm fetus (Figs. 10-14, 10-16, 10-24, and 10-25), and extends about 1-2 mm beyond the zone of the bony trabeculae of endochondral ossification. After the 250 mm fetus, the extent of endochondral and subperiosteal ossifications is the same (Fig. 10-26), and at term occupies three-fourth of the length of the metacarpal bones.

Before the fetal period starts, intramembranous ossification of the tip of cartilaginous distal phalanx is first seen (Fig. 10-5). The osteoblasts of the perichondral zone of the tip of the cartilaginous phalanx start to lay down a thick membranous bony lamella. The tuberosity of the distal phalanx is formed by the membranous bony trabeculae on the exterior of the subperiosteal cap in the 40 mm (Fig. 10-6). By the 60 mm fetus, endochondral ossification is first observed in the distal extremity of the distal phalanx (Figs. 10-13 and 10-28). After the 120 mm fetus, endochondral and subperiosteal ossification proceeds in only one direction, just proximally (Fig. 10-29). These findings demonstrate that intramembranous ossification, calcification, and endochondral ossification start at the tip of the distal phalanx instead of at the center of the shaft as is the case in the other long bone. A primary bone collar of the proximal phalanges is first noted in the 40 mm fetus, the latest being the fifth proximal phalanx. By the 60 mm fetus, endochondral ossification of the middle phalanx is observed (Fig. 10-13).

Cartilage canals of the carpal bones are first seen in the scaphoid and trapezium bones in the 70 mm fetus (Fig. 10-15) and in all carpal bones in the 90 and 100 mm fetuses (Figs. 10-17 and 10-18).

Cartilagenous sesamoids of the thumb are first found in the 40 mm fetus (Fig. 10-27). Accessory triangulare appears in the 60 mm fetus at the site distal to the developing articular disc (Fig. 10-12). The centrale makes its appearance as precartilage at the space adjacent to the scaphoid, trapezoid, and hamate in the 30 mm fetus (Fig. 10-4). By the 50 mm fetus, the scaphocentral fusion begins and in the 70 mm fetus it is complete, so that the centrale is no longer distinguishable (Fig. 10-15).

Homogenous interzones are present in each joint of the hand by the 20 mm embryo or later (Fig. 10-3). The homogenous interzone is differentiated into a three-layered interzone with two chondrogenous layers and an intermediate layer by the 35 mm fetus (Fig. 10-7). In the early developmental stage, the intermediate layer of interzone consists of a zone which is 3-4 elongated cell thick, but in a later phase the cells are converted into chondroblasts and incorporated into the chondrogenous layer.

The primitive joint cavities of the radiocarpal and midcarpal joints are first seen in the three-layered interzone as a narrow cleft around the periphery in the 40 mm fetus (Fig. 10-8) and are complete in the 50 and 60 mm fetuses (Figs. 10-9 and 10-12). By the 70 mm fetus, the radioscaphoid, radiolunate and ulnotriquetral joints in later stage form a single continuous joint cavity of the wrist (Fig. 10-15). By the 50 mm fetus, the pisotriquetral joint cavity appears independent and separates from the wrist joint cavity by a thin cellular strand in the 100 mm fetus. In many of the specimens, the pisotriquetral joint cavity is in communication with the ulnar part of the wrist joint cavity (Figs. 10-10, 10-18, and 10-19). A synovial membrane is observed to have the vascular invasion in a 50 mm fetus (Fig. 10-10), formation of the synovial folds by the 60 mm fetus (Fig. 10-12), and the collagenous fibers in the 100 mm fetus. The prestyloid recess, which appears in the 60 mm fetus (Fig. 10-14) and enlarges in the 120 mm fetus, is found to have vascular synovial villi within the wall.

In the 30 mm fetus, the anlage of the articular disc is present as a mesenchymal cells occupying the area between the ulnar styloid process and medial margin of the radius (Fig. 10-4). Progressing development of the radius, ulna, and carpal bones facilitates the definition of the disc area (Figs. 10-10, 10-14, and 10-20). By the 100 mm fetus, the articular disc is composed of densely arranged fibroblasts and general shapes almost similar to those of an adult (Fig. 10-21). By 110 mm fetus, the fibroblasts in the central zone of the articular disc are presented as oval profiles with a few short cell processes, whereas dorsal and palmar margins are presented as elongated cells. During the next 150 mm up to the 260 mm fetus, the central zone of the articular disc is composed of the intercrossed bundles of the collagenous fibers and populated by oval fibroblasts. The palmar and dorsal margins of the articular disc are constituted of parallel fascicules of the collagenous fibers with blood vessels and elongated fibroblasts. No fibrocartilage, however, can be found within it throughout this study (Fig. 10-22).

The anlagen of the radiocarpal and collateral ligaments are present as cellular condensations around many joints before cavities and, in some cases, before three-layered interzones appear. By the 40 mm fetus, the palmar radiocarpal ligament is shown to have distinct attachment to the lunate. Collateral ligaments of the radiocarpal and midcarpal joints are present as cellular condensations around many joints before cavities. By the 50 mm fetus, radiocarpal, collateral, and intercarpal ligaments are observed (Fig. 10-10). The primordium of tendons is first identified in the 30 mm fetus. The flexor digitorum profundus and sublimis can be seen in the 50 mm fetus. Synovial sheath formation has commenced by the 40 mm fetus, and completed by the 100 mm fetus (Figs. 10-18, 10-19, and 10-23).

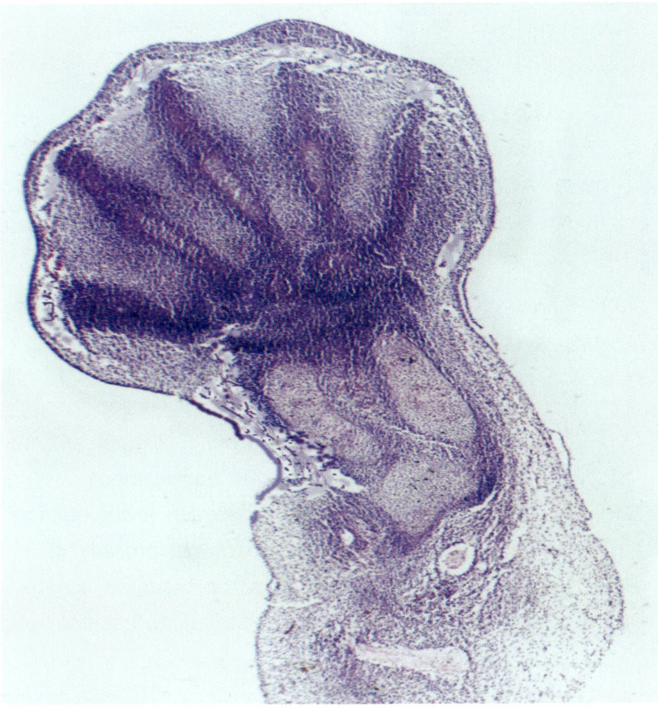

Fig. 10-1. Frontal section through the hand from a 10 mm embryo, showing developing cartilage models of forearm and hand. The radius, ulna, and humerus are distinguishable as skeletal blastema. The carpal region is formed by a dense mass of blastema. The metacarpal region shows early centers of the skeletal blastema.

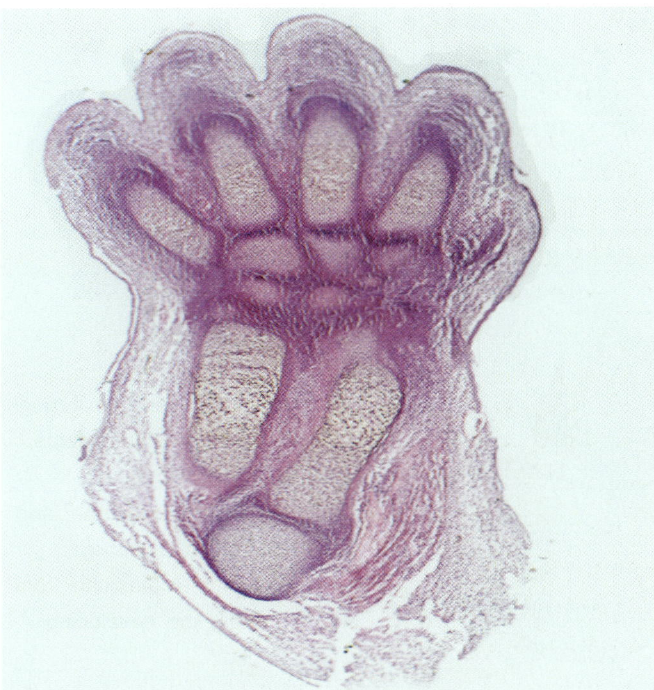

Fig. 10-2. Frontal section through the hand from a 14 mm embryo, showing chondrification of the carpal bones, radius, and ulna. The carpal elements of the proximal and distal rows are chondrified, and are separated from each other. The phalangeal region of the blastema is still undifferentiated.

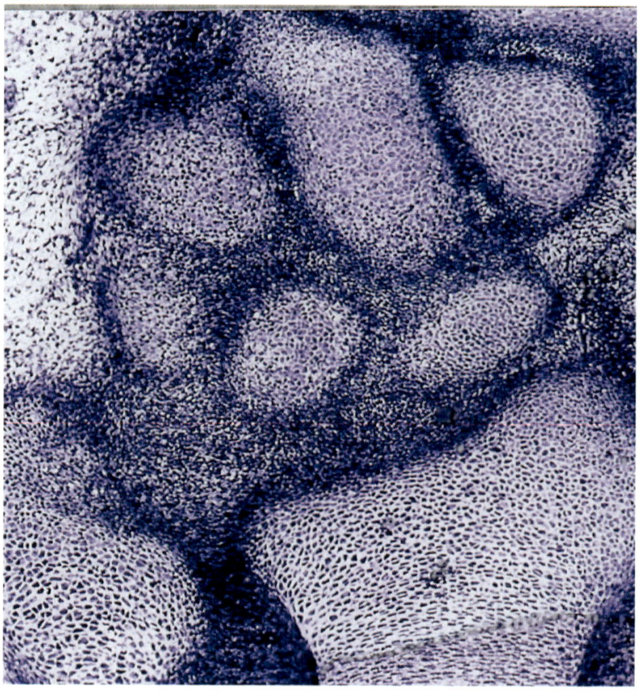

Fig. 10-3. Frontal section through the hand from a 20 mm embryo, showing the homogenous interzone between lower ends of radius and styloid process of ulna. Note the triquetral, lunate, scaphoid, trapetium, capitate, and hamate.

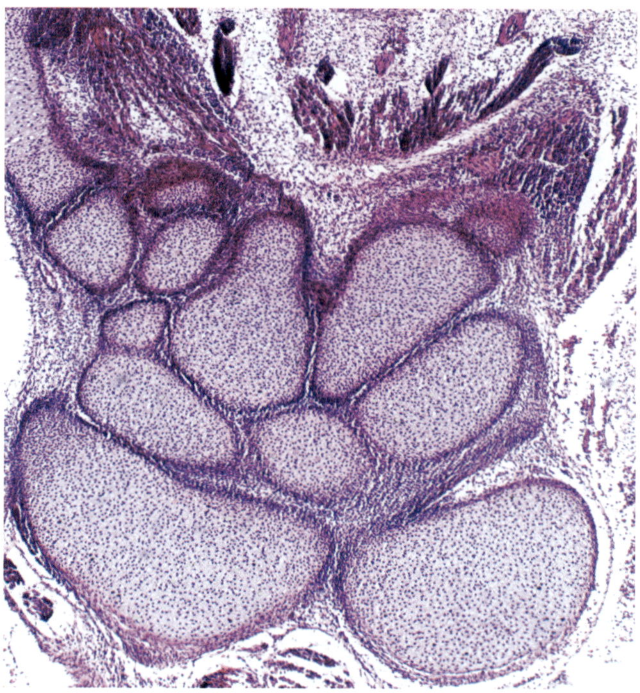

Fig. 10-4. Frontal section through the hand from a 30 mm fetus, showing the homogenous interzone of the radiocarpal and intercarpal joints. Scaphoid separated by the interzone from centrale. Note the developing articular disc.

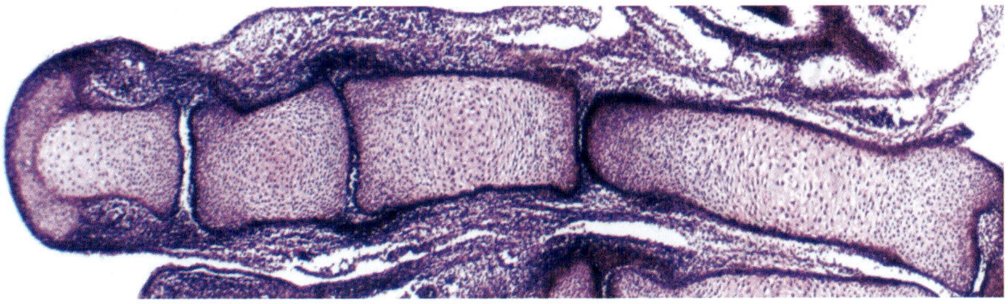

Fig. 10-5. Sagittal section through the finger from a 28 mm embryo, showing early ossification at the tip of distal phalanx. Membranous ossification at the tip of the distal phalanx is shown.

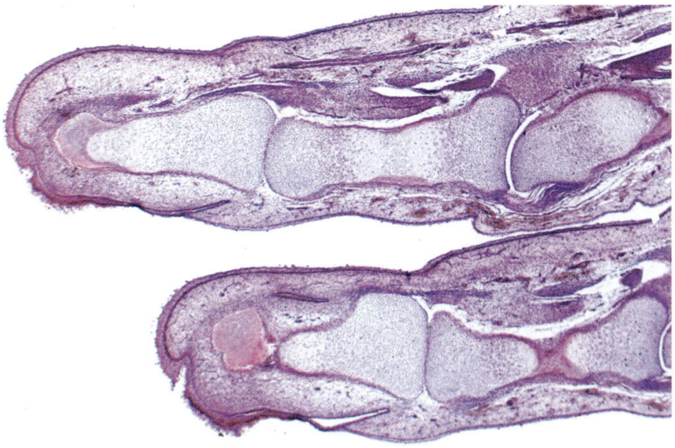

Fig. 10-6. Sagittal section through the 3rd and 4th fingers from a 40 mm fetus, showing membranous ossification at the tip of the distal phalanx.

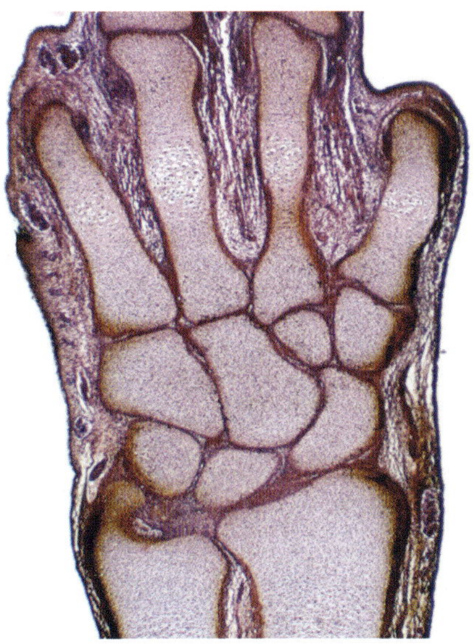

Fig. 10-7. Frontal section through the hand from a 35 mm fetus, showing bone collar and hypertrophied cartilage cells of the metacarpals of the 2nd, 3rd, 4th, and 5th fingers. Three-layered interzones of the radiocarpal and intercarpal joints are observed. The ulnar styloid process articulates with the triquetral via an independent joint cavity.

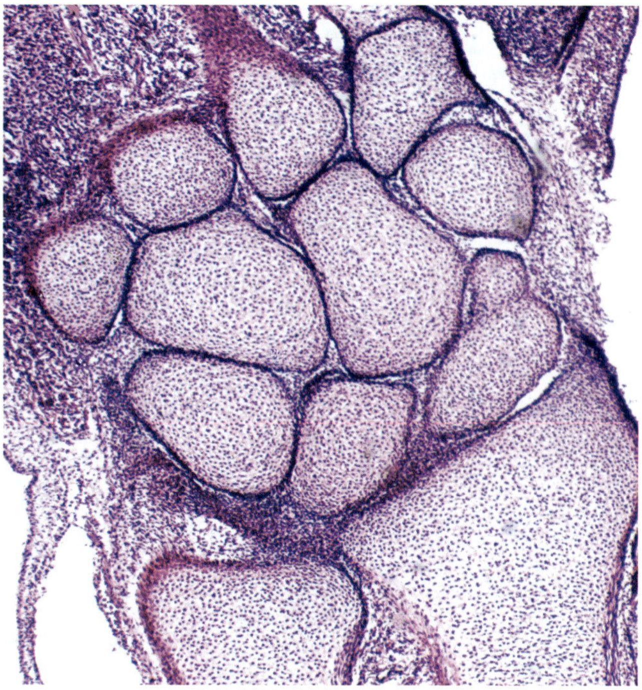

Fig. 10-8. Frontal section through the hand of a 40 mm fetus, showing beginning cavitation of early radiocarpal and midcarpal joints. Note the cartilaginous fusion between the scaphoid and centrale.

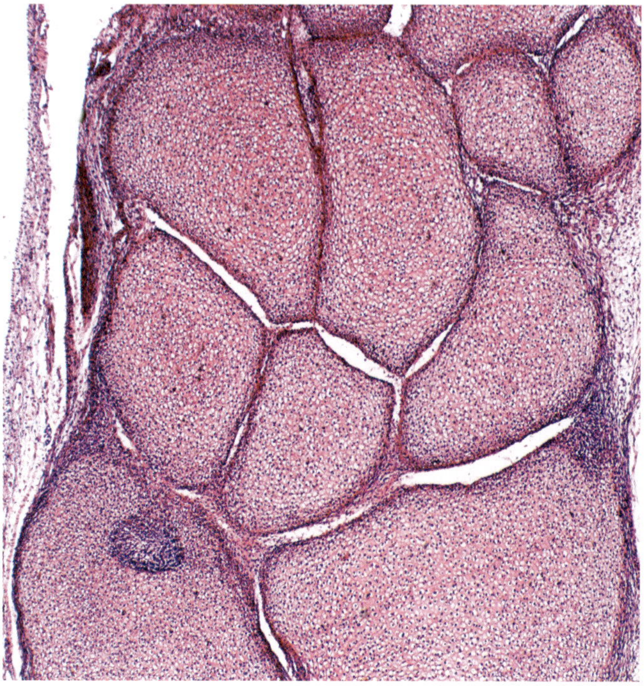

Fig. 10-9. Frontal section through the hand from a 50 mm fetus, showing complete formation of the intercarpal joints. The ulnar styloid process is in contact with the triquetrum. An incipient ulnocarpal cavity is present.

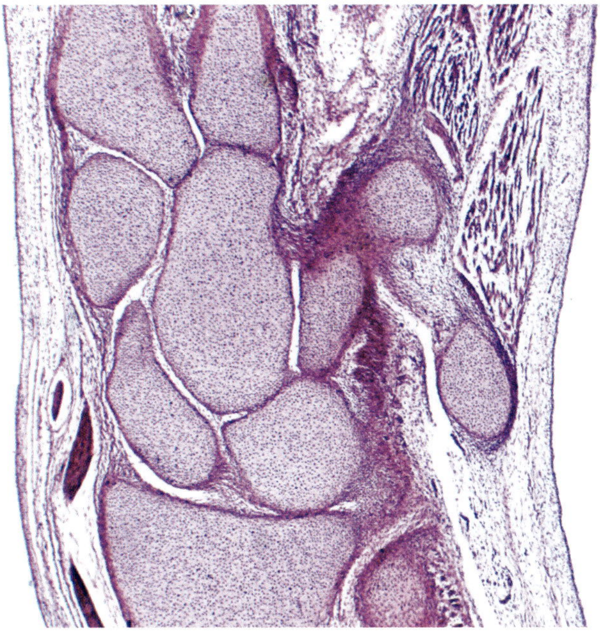

Fig. 10-10. Frontal section through the hand from a 50 mm fetus to show the pisotriquetral joint cavity which extends proximally into the developing articular disc. The intercarpal ligament between scaphoid and lunate is shown. Note the blood vessels on the synovial surface.

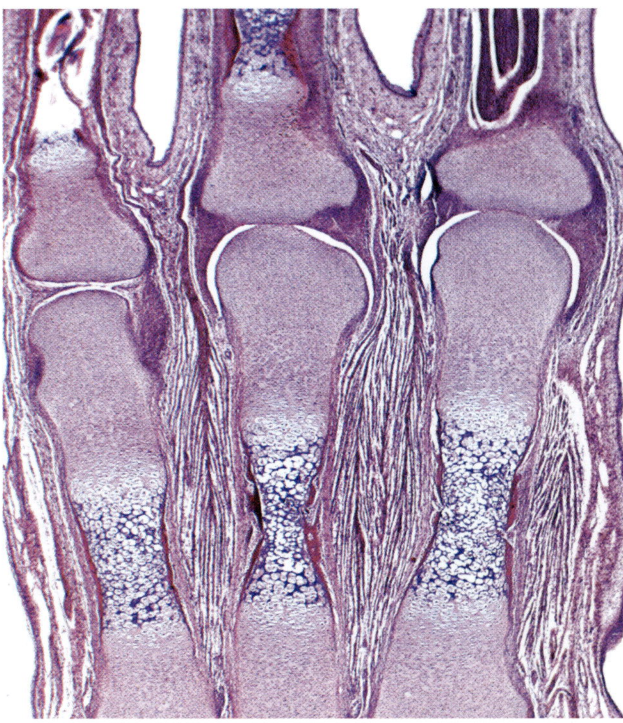

Fig. 10-11. Frontal section through the hand from a 50 mm fetus to show endochondral and subperiosteal bone formation of the 2nd, 3rd, and 4th metacarpal and proximal phalangeal bones.

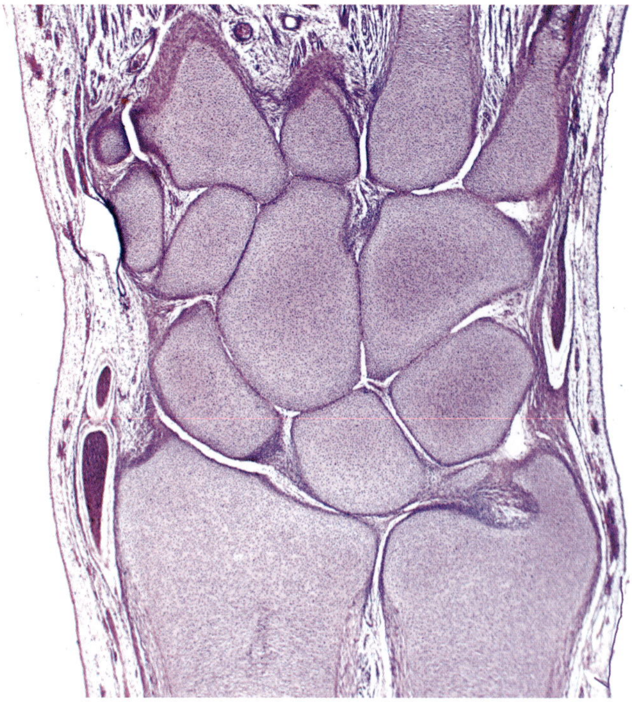

Fig. 10-12. Frontal section through the hand from a 60 mm fetus to show the complete formation of carpal joints. The articular disc and intercarpal ligaments are seen. A cartilaginous triangularen (intermedium antebrachii) lies in the loose mesenchyme distal to the developing triangular articular disc. Vascular synovial folds project for the first time into intercarpal joint cavities.

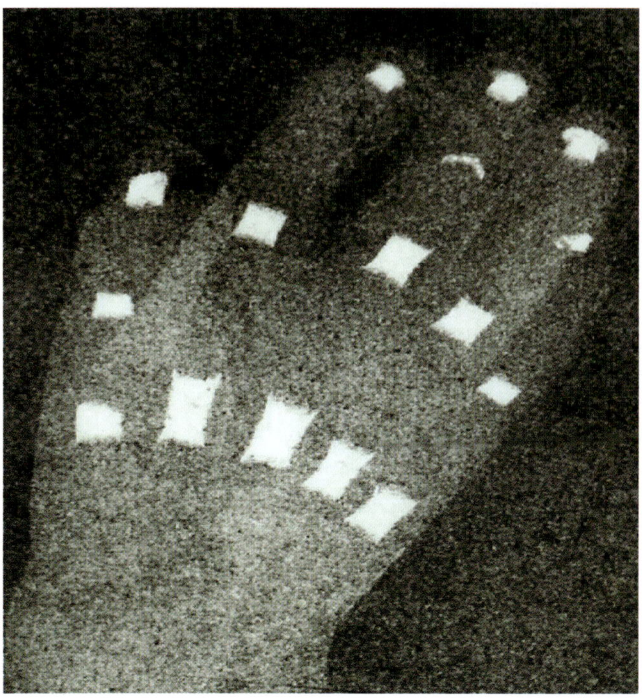

Fig. 10-13. Roentgenogram of the hand of a 60 mm fetus after silver impregnation to show the ossification centers of the metacarpal and phalangeal bones.

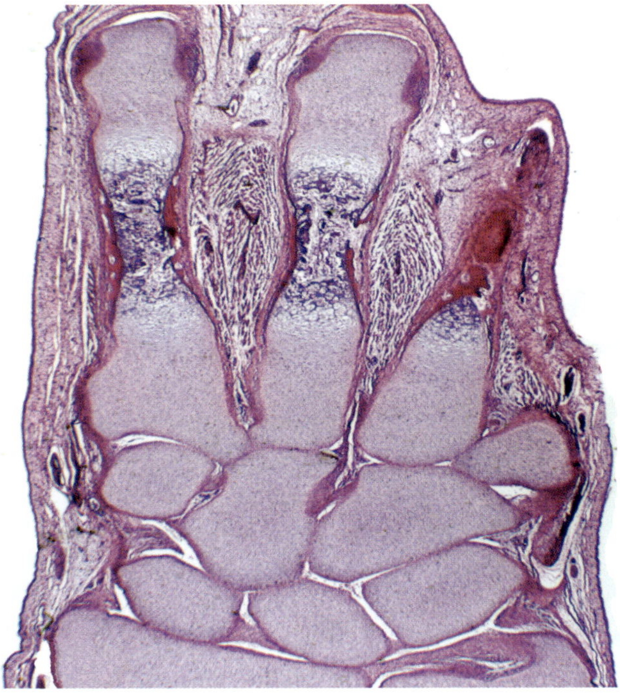

Fig. 10-14. Frontal section through the hand from a 60 mm fetus to show multiple invasion of bone collar of the metacarpal bones by the periosteal bud. The prestyloid recess develops as an extension of the wrist joint cavity delaminating the articular disc from the styloid process and articular disc.

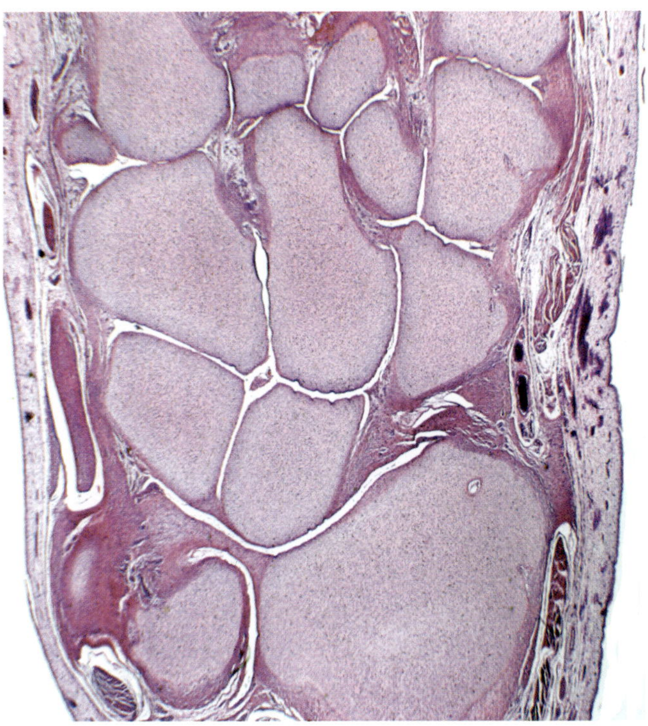

Fig. 10-15. Frontal section through the hand from a 70 mm fetus to show the articular disc attached to the radius, and L-shaped radioulnar cavity. The radiolunate and radiotriquetral joints form a single continuous joint cavity. The intercarpal ligaments are seen. Cartilage canals are first seen in scaphoid and trapezium bones.

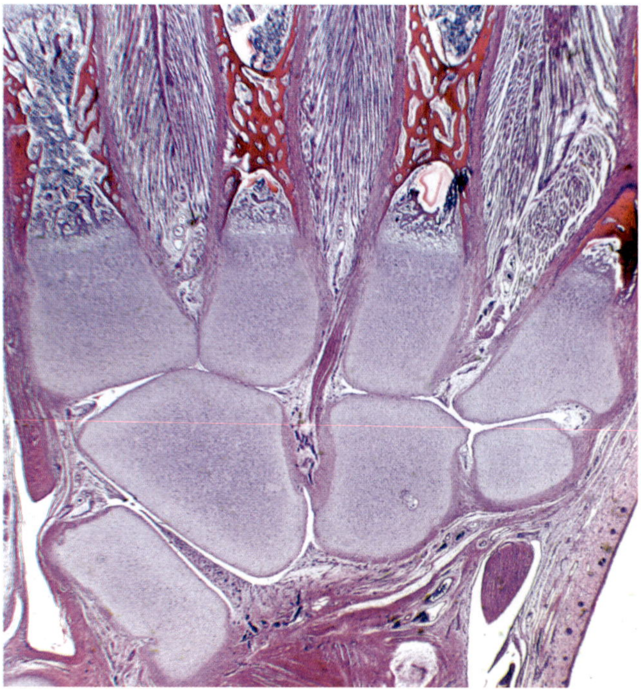

Fig. 10-16. Frontal section through the hand from a 90 mm fetus to show endochondral and subperiosteal ossification of the four metacarpal bones. As endochondral ossification proceeds proximally and distally, periosteal bone formation extends proximally beyond the level of the endochondral ossification.

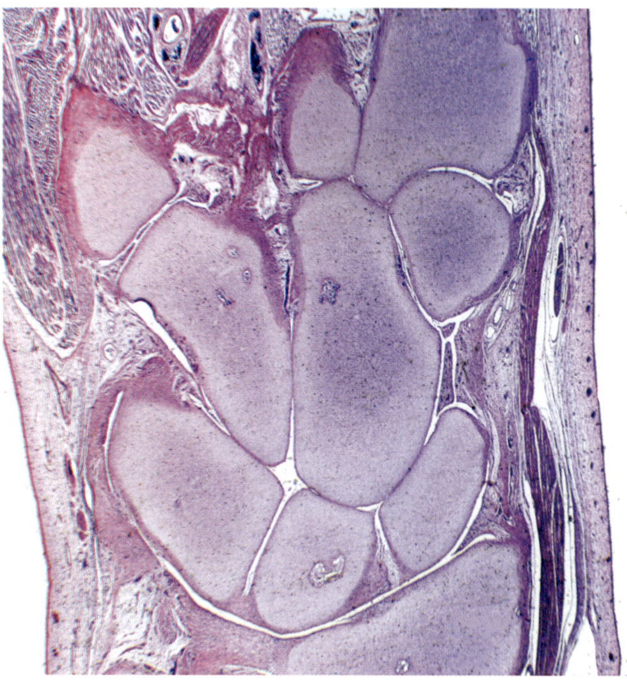

Fig. 10-17. Frontal section through the hand from a 90 mm fetus to show cartilage canals in the lunate, triquetral, capitate, and hamate bones.

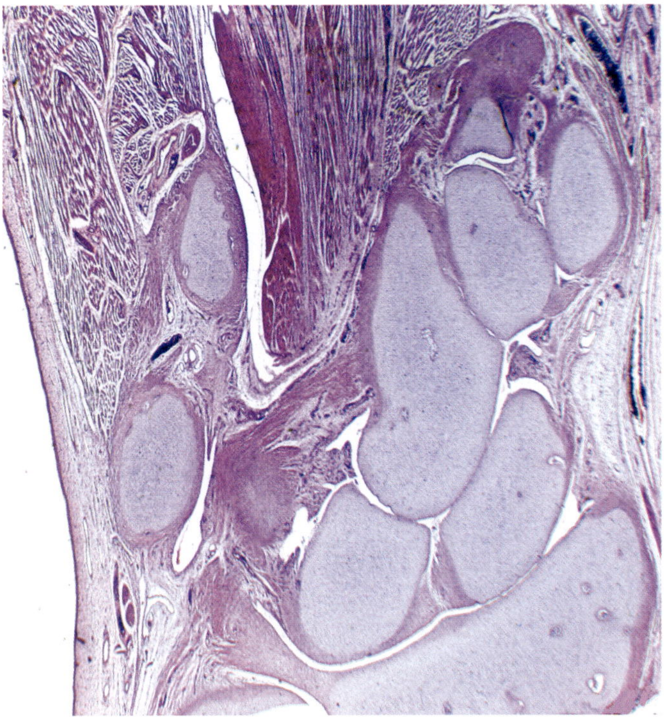

Fig. 10-18. Frontal section through the hand from a 100 mm fetus to show articular disc and intercarpal ligaments. The pisotriquetral joint cavity extends proximally, close to the periphery of the developing articular disc. Cartilage canals are seen in all carpal bones.

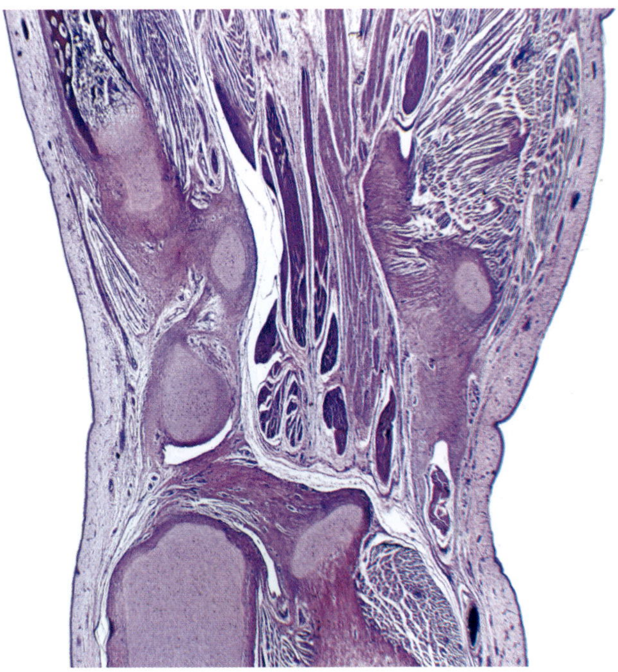

Fig. 10-19. Frontal section through the hand from a 100 mm fetus to show tendons of flexor digitorum sublimis and profundus, and lumbricals. The pisotriquetral cavity extends proximally into a relationship with the developing articular disc.

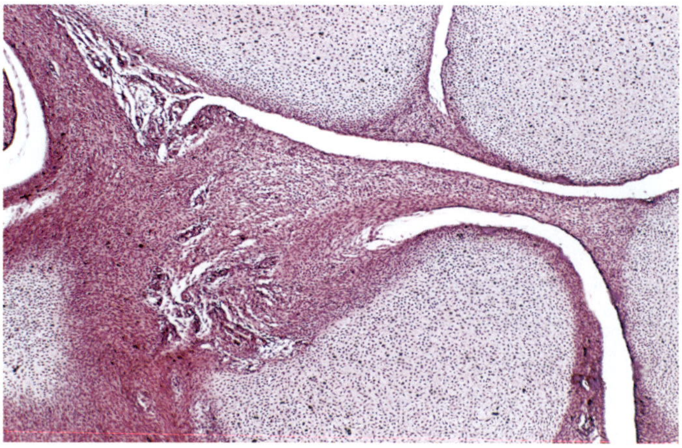

Fig. 10-20. Frontal section of the wrist joint from a 70 mm fetus to show the fibroblast, collagenous fibers, and blood vessels of the developing articular disc.

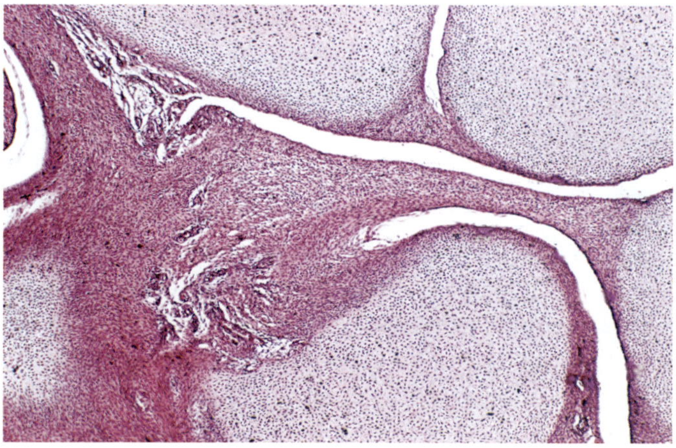

Fig. 10-21. Frontal section from a 100 mm fetus to show the articular disc. The ulnar and carpal surfaces are composed of condensed collagen fibers and they are more cellular than the central part. In a distal direction the disc continues into the tendon sheath of the extensor carpi ulnaris.

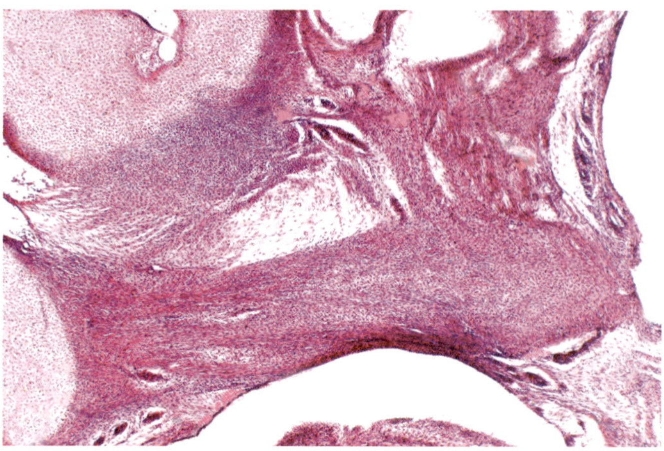

Fig. 10-22. Frontal section of wrist joint of a 200 mm fetus to show the developing articular disc. The central part of the disc showing the intercrossed bundles of collagen fibers that run in radioulnar and dorsopalmar directions.

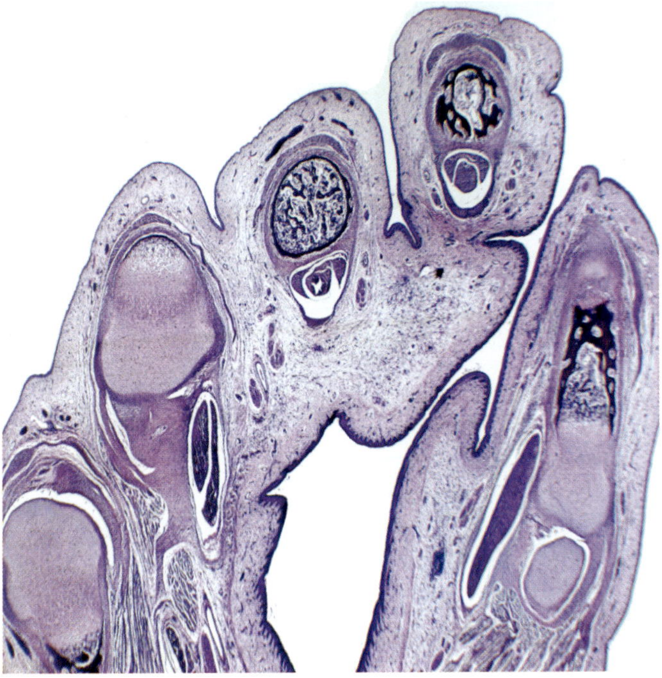

Fig. 10-23. Horizontal section of the phalangeal bones from a 130 mm fetus showing the endochondral trabeculae with a periosteally formed shell. The tendons of the flexor digitorum superficialis and profundus are clearly separated. Nerves, vessels, and lumbrical muscles can be recognized.

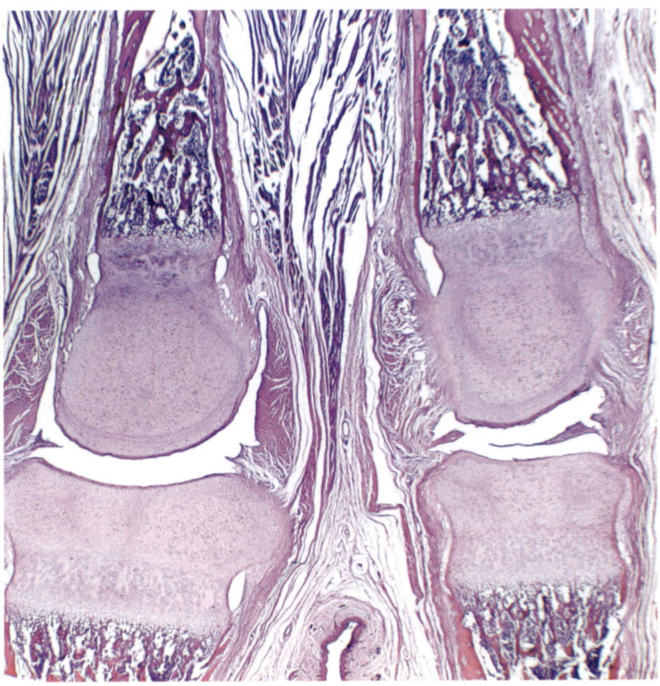

Fig. 10-24. Frontal section of the metacarpal and proximal phalangeal bones from a 180 mm fetus to show ossification. The extents of endochondral and subperiosteal ossification are the same.

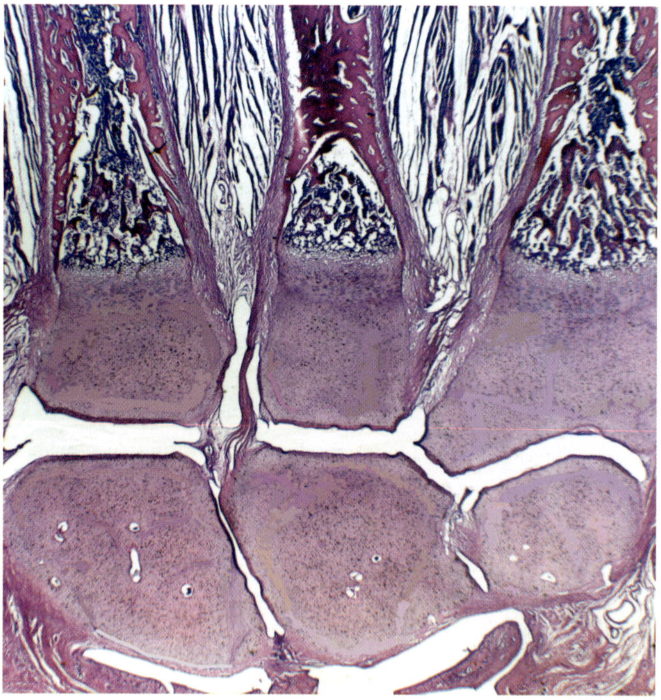

Fig. 10-25. Frontal section of the hand in a 200 mm fetus to show the cartilage canals in trapezoid, capitate, and hamate bones.

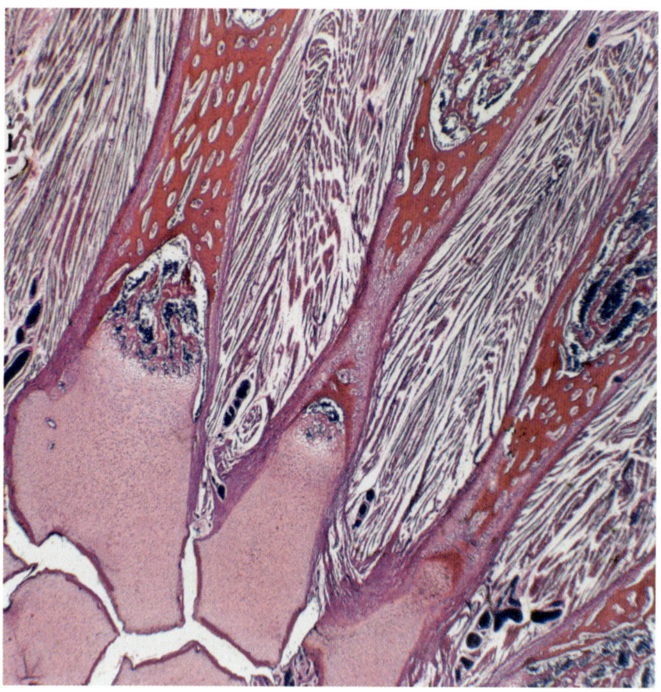

Fig. 10-26. Frontal section through the hand from a 250 mm fetus to show endochondral ossification of the metacarpal bones. Note the cartilage canals in the base of the metacarpal bones. The extents of the endochondral and subperiosteal ossification are almost the same and occupy three-fourth of the length of the metacarpal bones.

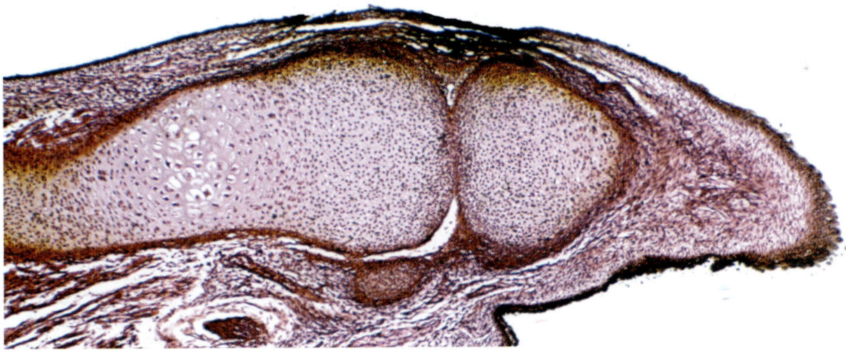

Fig. 10-27. Sagittal section through the thumb from a 40 mm fetus, showing the metacarpophalngeal sesamoid. Note the chondrification beginning in cellular condensation.

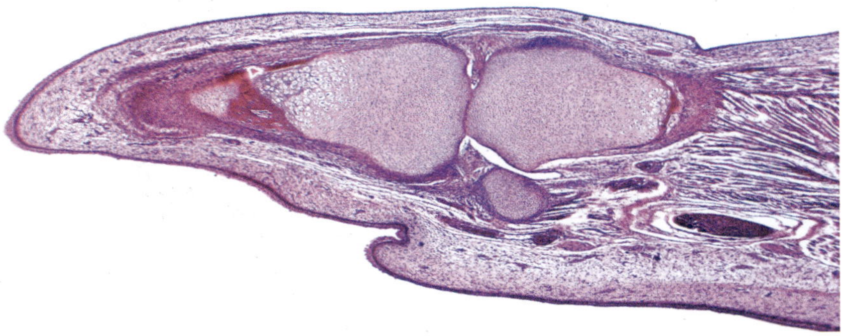

Fig. 10-28. Sagittal section through the thumb from a 60 mm fetus, showing the metacarpophalangeal sesamoid. Note the relation of muscle fibers to the sesamoid.

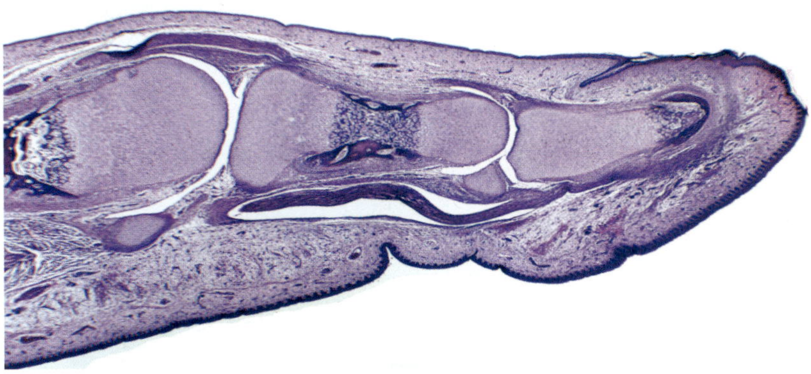

Fig. 10-29. Sagittal section through the thumb of a 120 mm fetus, showing the metacarpophalangeal and interphalangeal sesamoids of the thumb.

References

Ahn HB, Yoon JR: The development of the articular disc of human distal radioulnar joint. *Korean J Phys Anthrop* 6: 73-93, 1993.

Corner EM: The morphology of the triangular cartilage of the wrist. *J Anat* 32: 272-277, 1898.

Gray DJ, Gardner E, O'Rahilly R: The prenatal development of the skeleton and joints of the human hand. *Am J Anat* 101: 169-224, 1957.

Lewis OJ: The development of the human wrist joint during the fetal period. *Anat Rec* 166: 499-516, 1969.

O'Rahilly R, Gardner E, Gray DJ: The skeletal developmenrt of the hand. *Clinical Orthopaedics* 13: 42-51, 1959.

Yoon JR, Bae CS, An KY: The prenatal development of the skeleton and joints of the human hand. *Chonnam Medical J* 23: 349-364, 1986.

The Development of the Sacroiliac Joint and Pevis

Chapter 11

The earlier studies on the development of the pelvis are largely concerned with observations on the developing skeletal elements. The skeleton of the ilium consists largely of condensed blastemal tissue of 9 to 12 mm embryos. The center of chondrification for the ilium, ischium, and pubis appears in the 22 to 25 mm embryos (Fig. 11-1). The acetabulum is somewhat deeper medially than laterally. This increase in depth is marked in 30 to 35 mm fetuses, and the pubis, iliac, and ischial cartilages clearly take part in the formation of the acetablum (Figs. 11-2 and 11-3).

The perichondral bone of the ilium in the vincity of the greater sciatic notch is seen in the 40 mm fetus (Fig. 11-4). In the 55 mm fetus, endochondral bone formation of the ilium is first noted. Ossification spreads in two directions, inferiorly toward the triradiate zone and anteriorly toward the anterior inferior iliac spine (Figs. 11-7 and 11-8). Later, ossification spreads laterally toward the acetabulum in the 100 to 120 mm fetuses (Fig. 11-10). By the 230 mm fetus, the center of ossification spreads laterally and inferiorly into the base of the acetabulum (Fig. 11-13). Ossification centers are first noted in the ischium in the 100 mm fetus and the pubis in the 120 mm fetus (Fig. 11-10). In the 260 mm fetus, ossification is almost complete in the body of ischium and pubis (Fig. 11-14).

The symphysis pubis is first seen as a mesenchymal condensation between the anlagen of the adjacent surfaces of the pubic bones in the 40 mm fetus (Figs. 11-5 and 11-6). In the 55 mm fetus, the interpubic disc is seen as a line in the upper part of the symphysis. The anlagen of the arcuate pubic and inferior pubic ligaments are present as cellular condensations around the symphysis (Figs. 11-7 and 11-9). The superior pubic and arcuate pubic ligaments are well defined in the 130 mm fetus (Fig. 11-11).

The development of the sacroiliac joint belongs to a rather neglected field of recent investigation. Much has been written concerning structure, function, and surgery of the sacroiliac joint, but little has been done on its development. Its cranial part is synarthrodial in nature. Its caudal part, corresponding to the auricular surfaces, has recently been classified as a synovial joint (Bowen and Cassidy, 1981).

In the 22 mm embryo, the interzone of the sacroiliac joint is homogenous and continuous with the perichondrium surrounding the cartilages (Fig. 11-1). The homogenous interzone is differentiated into a three-layered interzone with two chondrogenous layers and an intermediate layer by the 35 mm fetus (Fig. 11-3). From there on, the development of the sacroiliac joint is quite different from that of other joints. By the 40 mm fetus, the primitive joint cavity is present at the caudal part of the sacroiliac joint (Fig. 11-4).

Cavitation at the caudal part proceeds very slowly during the third month. By 55 mm fetus, the sacroiliac joint is seen only as a very small cavity which is located in the caudal part of the joint. Its middle and cranial parts are synarthrodial in nature (Fig. 11-8). The articular cavity is still very small and is found in the caudal part of the joint in the 90 mm fetus (Fig. 11-10). By the 160 mm fetus, the definitive joint cavity is still very incomplete, bridged by a few fibrous interarticular bands in its midportion only (Fig. 11-12). The iliac joint surface is covered by a thick layer of fibrous tissue, but the sacral side is covered with hyaline cartilage in the 260 mm fetus. Interarticular bands are present throughout the fetal life (Fig. 11-14).

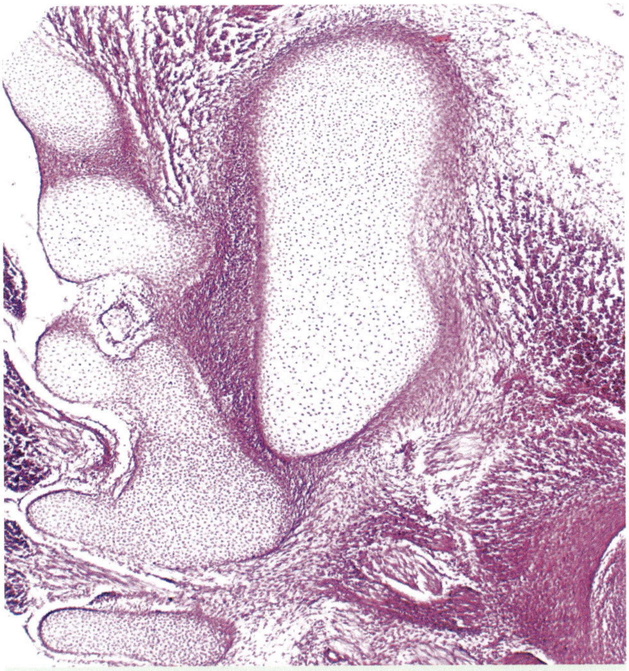

Fig. 11-1. Frontal section through the midportion of the pelvis from a 22 mm embryo, showing the homogenous interzone of the sacroiliac joint. The sacral and iliac cartilages are separated by a mass of mesenchymal cells.

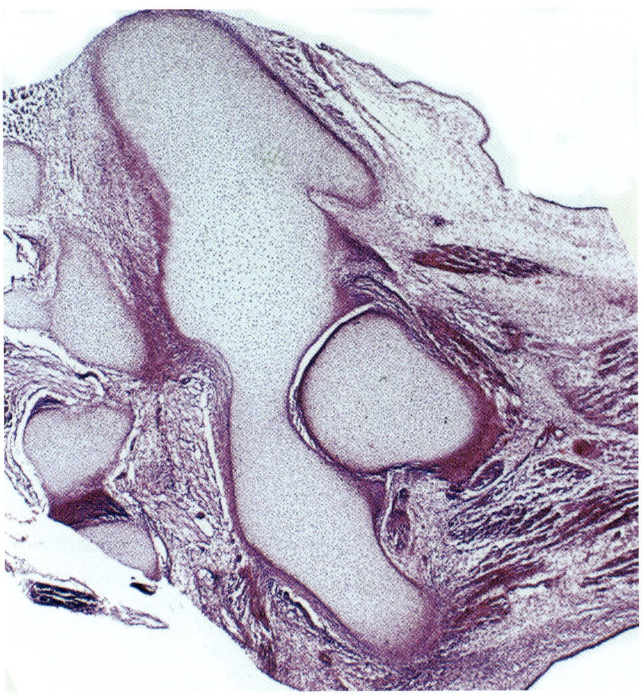

Fig. 11-2. Frontal section through the midportion of the pelvis in a 30 mm fetus, showing acetabulum. The pubic, iliac, and ischial cartilages clearly enter into the formation of the acetabulum.

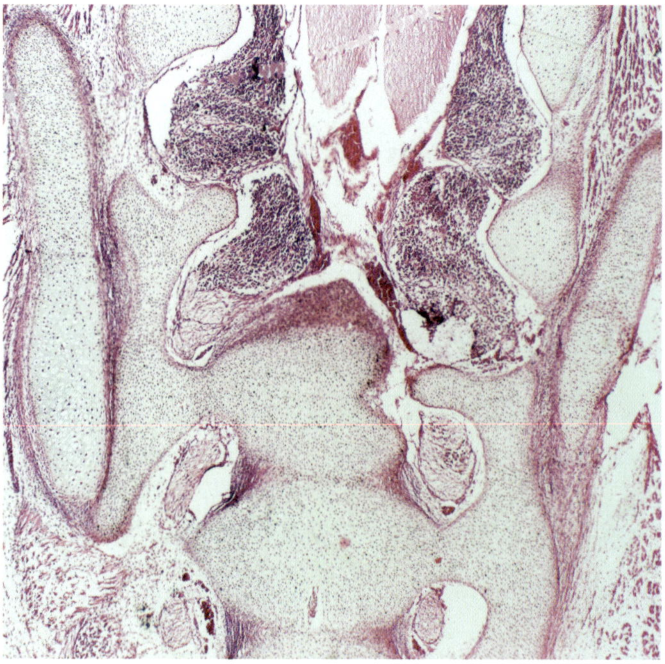

Fig. 11-3. Frontal section through the midportion of the sacroiliac joint of a 35 mm fetus, showing the three-layered interzone of the sacroiliac joint. Note the spinal nerves and ganglia in the sacral foramina.

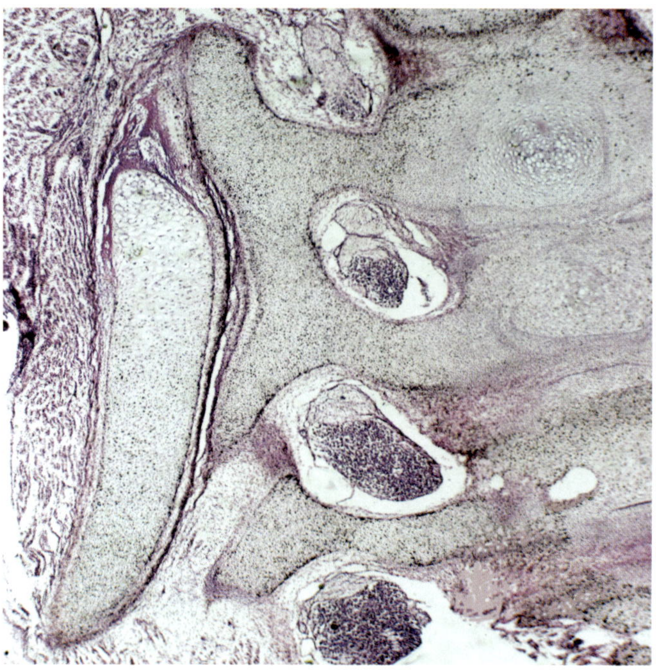

Fig. 11-4. Frontal section through the midportion of the sacroiliac joint from a the 40 mm fetus to show the beginning cavitation at the caudal part of the interzone. The perichondral bone formation is clearly visible on the medial and lateral aspects of the ilium.

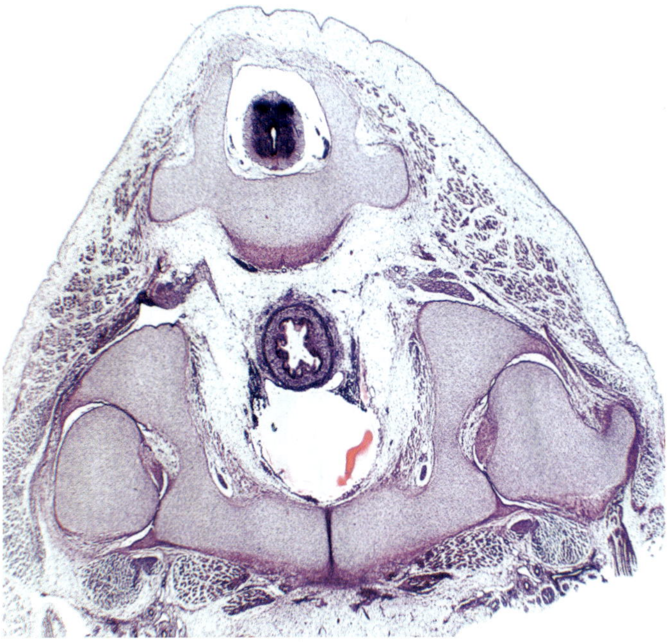

Fig. 11-5. Transverse section through the part of symphysis pubis from a 40 mm fetus to show the cartilaginous pelvis. The superior ramus of the pubis and the ilium are one cartilaginous anlage.

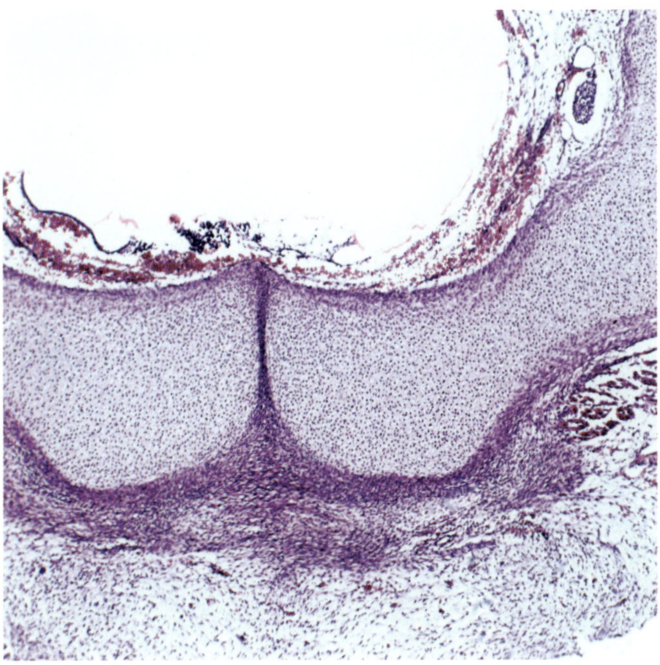

Fig. 11-6. Transverse section through the part of the superior ramus of the pubis from a 40 mm fetus, showing pubic symphysis. The arcuate pubic ligament, together with the interpubic disc, are observed as mesenchymal condensation.

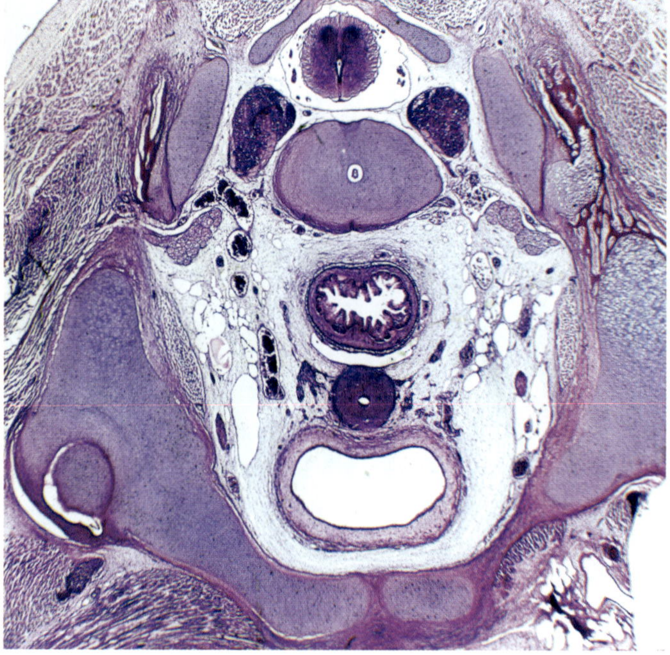

Fig. 11-7. Transverse section through the cranial portion of a sacroiliac joint from a 55 mm fetus, showing the advanced bone formation of the ilium. The cavitation does not reach into this zone. Ossification spreads in two directions, inferiorly toward the acetabulum and anteriorly toward anterior inferior iliac spine.

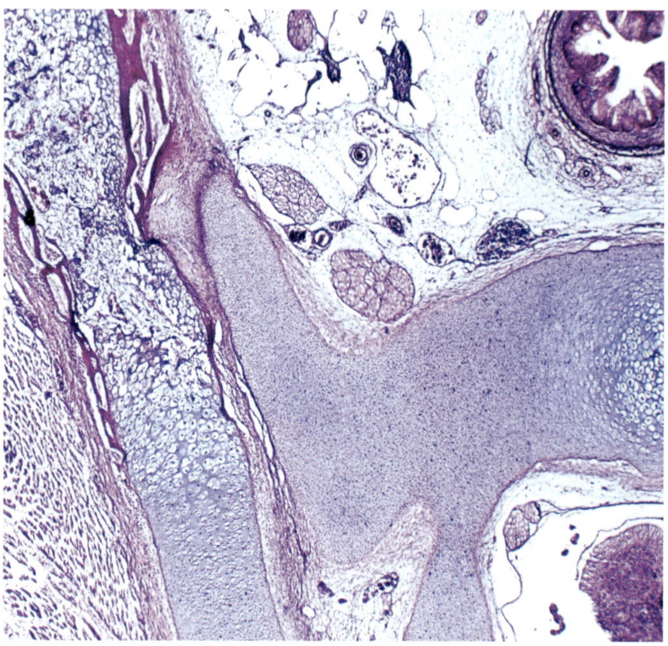

Fig. 11-8. Transverse section through the caudal part of the sacroiliac joint in a 55 mm fetus, showing formation of the synovial joint. The cavitation of the sacroiliac joint is very small and is found only in the caudal portion of the joint.

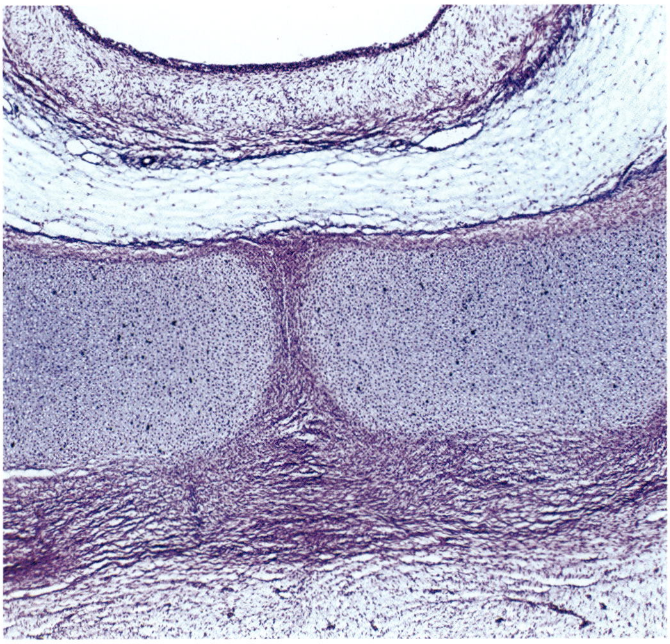

Fig. 11-9. Transverse section through the part of the pubic symphysis from a 55 mm fetus, showing the interpubic disc. The arcuate pubic ligament is well defined. The interpubic disc is seen in the upper part of the joint as a fine line.

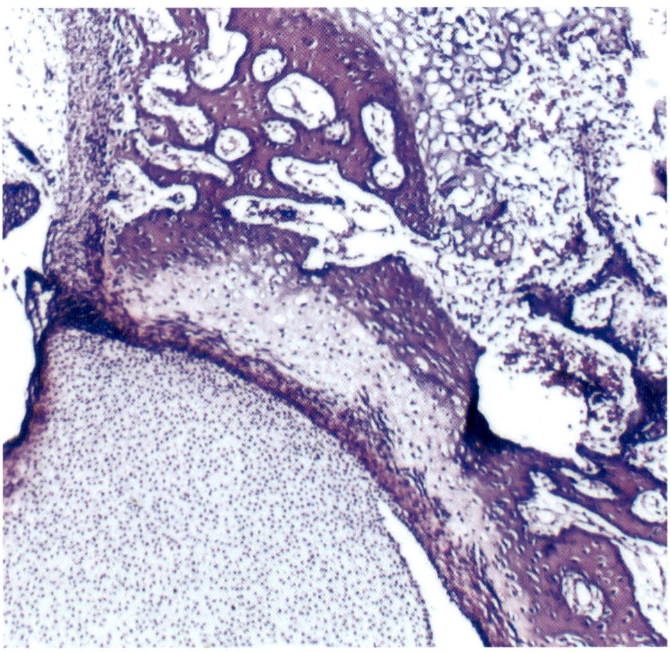

Fig. 11-10. Sagittal section through the midportion of the sacroiliac joint of a 100 mm fetus to show cavitation of the synovial joint and synarthrosis. Cavitation in the sacroiliac joint appears at the caudal part but does not reach its full extent.

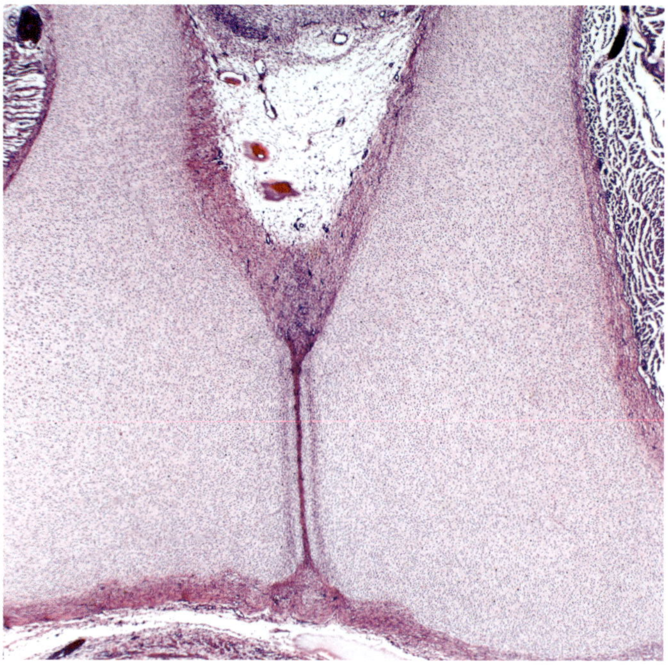

Fig. 11-11. Frontal section through the midportion of the pubic symphysis from a 130 mm fetus, showing a well-defined superior and arcuate pubic ligaments. The interpubic disc of the collagenous bundle is interposed between the adjacent surfaces of the pubic bones.

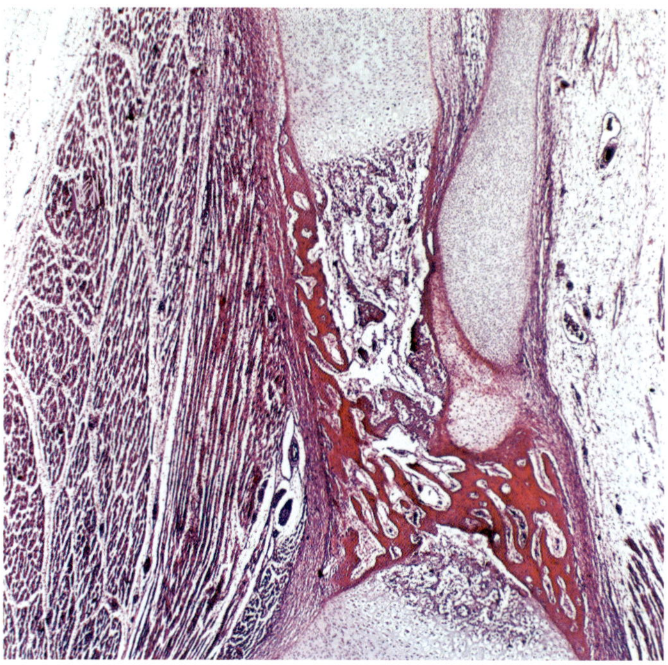

Fig. 11-12. Frontal section through the middle of the acetabulum from a 160 mm fetus to show endochondral ossification and subperiosteal bone formation. The definitive articular cavity of the sacroiliac joint is still very incomplete.

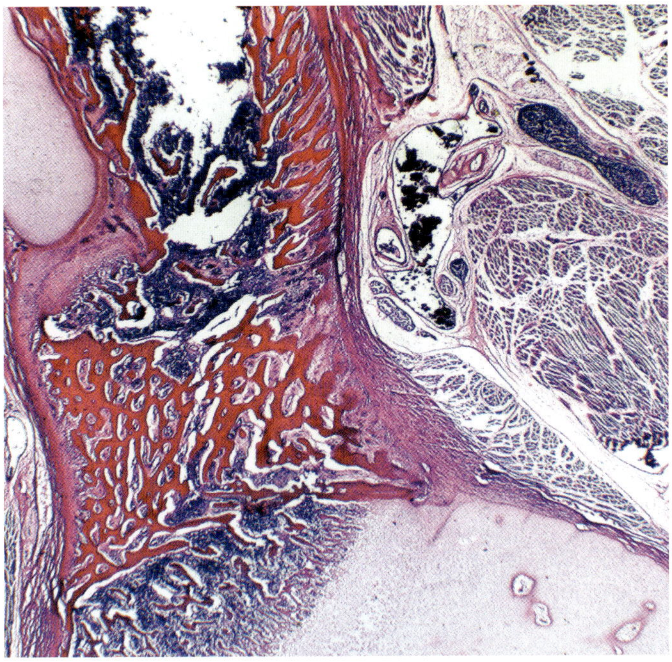

Fig. 11-13. Frontal section through the midportion of the acetabulum from a 230 mm fetus to show endochondral ossification and subperiosteal bone formation. Ossification of the innominate bone has reached the acetabular fossa and separates acetabulum from triradiate cartilage. The articular cavity of the sacroiliac joint is still very incomplete.

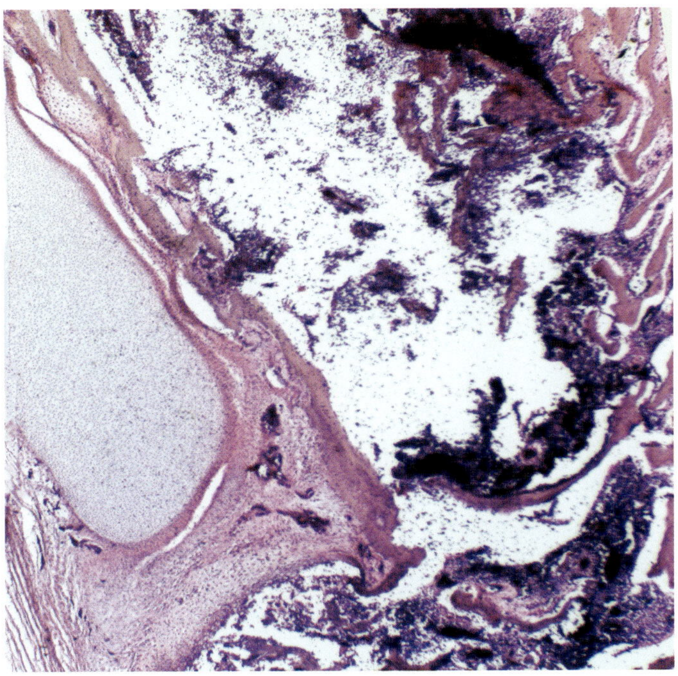

Fig. 11-14. Frontal section through the caudal and midportions of the sacroiliac joint from a 260 mm fetus to show a complete cavity, bridged by a few thin strands in its midportion only. The iliac articular cartilage is covered by a thick layer of fibrous tissue, but the sacral side is covered with hyaline cartilage.

References

Bowen V, Cassidy JD: Macroscopic and microscopic anatomy of the sacroiliac joint from the embryonic life until the eighth decade. *Spine* 6: 620-628, 1981.

Frances CL: Appearance of centers of ossification in human pelvis before birth. *AJR* 65: 778-783, 1951.

Gardner E, Gray DJ: Prenatal development of the hip joint. *Am J Anat* 87: 163-211, 1950.

Laurenson RD: The primary ossification of the human ilium. *Anat Rec* 148: 209-217, 1964.

Schunke GB: The anatomy and development of the sacroiliac joint in man. *Anat Rec* 72: 313-331, 1938.

The Development of the Hip Joint

Chapter 12

The skeletal blastema appears in the fore-limb bud as a diffuse condensation of the mesenchyme in the 7 mm embryo, and is complete by as far as the hand plate in the 9 mm embryo, while that of the hind-limb bud appears a little later, but is distinct by the 9 mm embryo (Haines, 1947). The skeleton of the hip joint consists largely of condensed blastemal tissue in the 13 mm embryo (Fig. 12-1). The acetabular fossa is indicated by the 20 to 22 mm embryos (Figs. 12-2 and 12-3). The femoral head and neck are present by the 22 to 25 mm embryos (Figs. 12-3 and 12-4). The fovea capitis femoris and both trochanters appear by the 35 to 40 mm fetuses (Figs. 12-7 and 12-8). Vascularization of epiphyseal cartilages of the proximal femur begins by the 50 to 55 mm fetuses (Fig. 12-11). Cartilage canals of the femur are first seen in the proximal epiphysis in the 70 mm fetus (Fig. 12-14), and in the distal epiphysis in the 80 mm fetus. A much more extensive vascularization of the femoral head and neck is noted in the 90 and 100 mm fetuses (Figs. 12-15, 12-16, and 12-17). By the 130 mm fetus, cartilage canals are numerous in the femoral head and acetabulum (Fig. 12-18).

Ossification centers are first seen in the femoral shaft in the 40 mm fetus (Fig. 12-8). As endochondral ossification of the femur proceeds proximally and distally, and growth zones become established, periosteal bone formation proceeds longitudinally until about 260 mm fetus. In the 40 mm fetus, endochondral bone formation of the ilium is first seen. Ossification spreads in two directions, inferiorly toward the triradiate cartilage and anteriorly toward the anterior inferior iliac spine in the 130 mm fetus (Fig. 12-19). Later, ossification spreads laterally toward the limbs in the 120 to 160 mm fetuses (Fig. 12-20). By the 230 mm fetus, the center of ossification of the ilium spreads laterally and inferiorly into the limbus (Figs. 12-22 and 12-23). At term, ossification of ilium has reached the acetabular fossa and separates acetabular cartilage from triradiate cartilages (Fig. 12-25).

As chondrification proceeds in the blastemal anlagen, the portion of the blastema between the femur and acetabulum remains unchondrified to form a primitive joint plate or homogenous interzone in the 12 to 20 mm embryos (Figs. 12-2 and 12-3). By the 22 mm embryo, a three-layered interzone is evident (Fig. 12-3). The initial joint cavity is present around the periphery of the joint in the 25 mm fetus, and is complete between the 35 and 40 mm fetuses (Figs. 12-6 and 12-9). The intermediate layer is continuous with the adjacent synovial mesenchyme in which capillaries appear by the 40 mm fetus (Figs. 12-6 and 12-10). By the 110mm fetus, villi are present, a few collagenous fibers become evident, and the distribution of blood vessels resembles that found in the adult (Fig. 12-17). The adipose tissue in the acetabular fossa is first seen in the 160 mm fetus (Fig. 12-21).

The primordia of the extraarticular capsule are found in the 25 mm embryo (Fig. 12-4). Fine collagenous fibers are present in this condensation in the 30 mm fetus (Fig. 12-5). Regional thickening of the capsule in the 60 mm fetus results from deposition of the collagenous fibers (Fig. 12-12).

The ligament of the head of the femur and acetabular labrum appear as cellular condensations in the 25 mm embryo (Fig. 12-4) and transverse acetabular ligament in the 35 mm fetus (Fig. 12-7). By the 60 mm fetus, the labrum near the acetabular notch is composed of numerous collagenous bundles and cells and is clearly demarcated from the adjacent hyaline cartilage (Fig. 12-13). Blood vessels in the ligament of the head of the femur are first seen in the 70 mm fetus (Fig. 12-14). By the 230 to 260 mm fetuses, many vessels pass up to the fovea capitis femoris, but relatively few enter the cartilage of the femoral head (Figs. 12-24 and 12-25).

Both the bursa iliopectinea and the subtendinous bursa of the obturator internus are observed in the 35 mm fetus (Fig. 12-7).

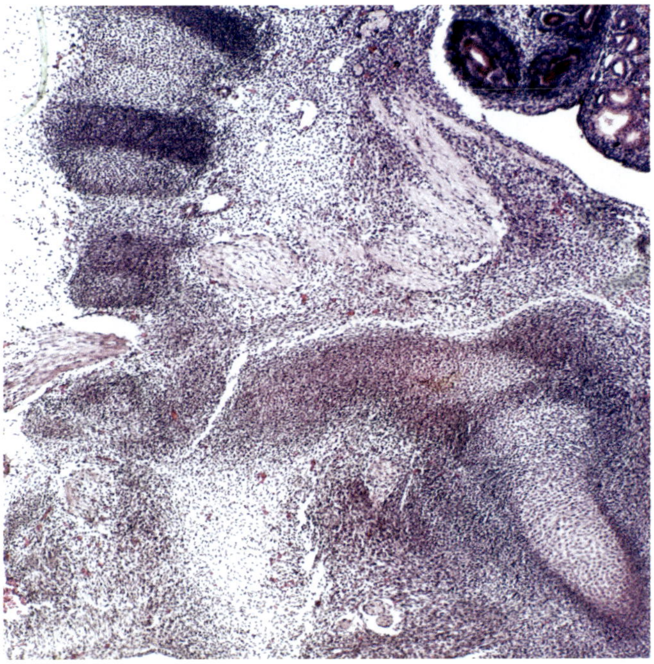

Fig. 12-1. Frontal section through the midportion of the hip joint in a 12 mm embryo to show the skeletal blastema of the lumbar vertebrae, pelvis, and femoral head. The cartilaginous primordia of the pevis and femoral head are separated by a blastemic condensation of mesenchymal tissue. Note the lumbar plexus between the lumbar vertebrae and pelvis.

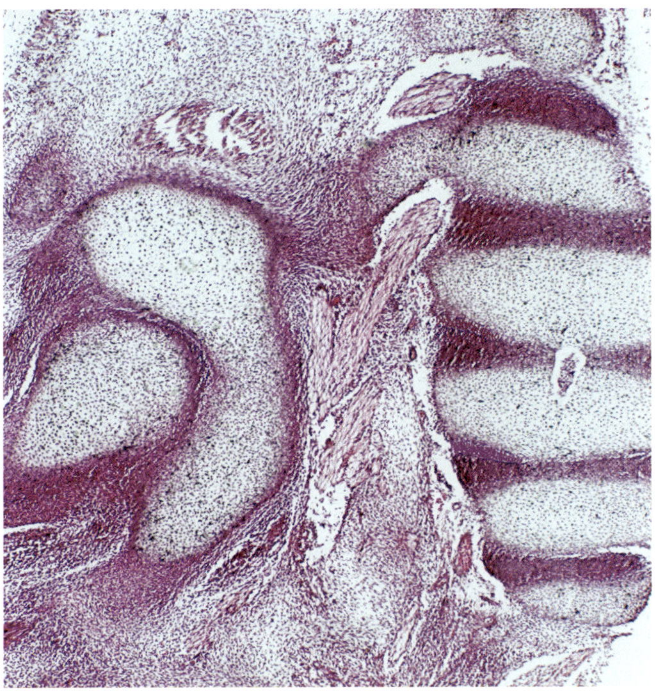

Fig. 12-2. Frontal section of the hip joint from a 20 mm embryo, showing the primordia of the acetabulum and the head of the femur. Between the lumbar vertebrae and the acetabulum, the lumbar plexus can be seen. Note the homogenous interzone between the acetabulum and the femoral head.

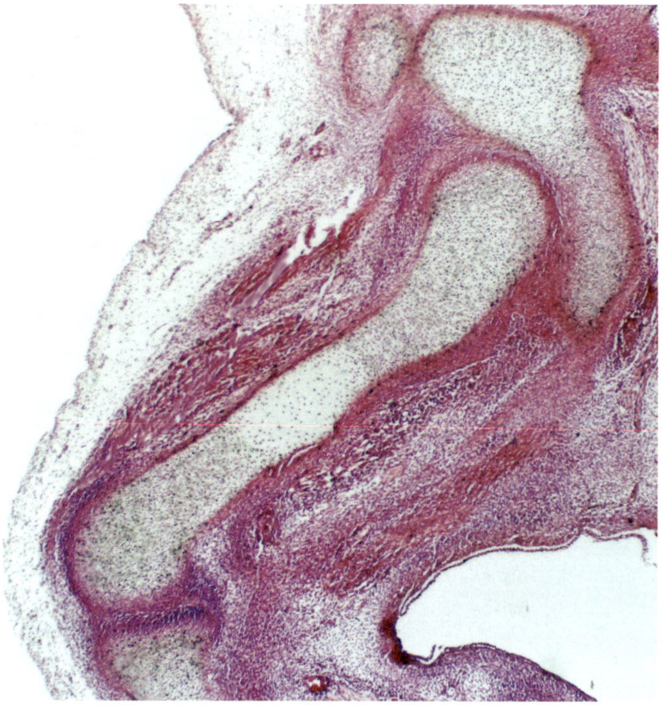

Fig. 12-3. Sagittal section of the hip joint from a 22 mm embryo, showing the three-layered interzone of the hip and knee joints. The head of the femur is rounded and the neck is constricted.

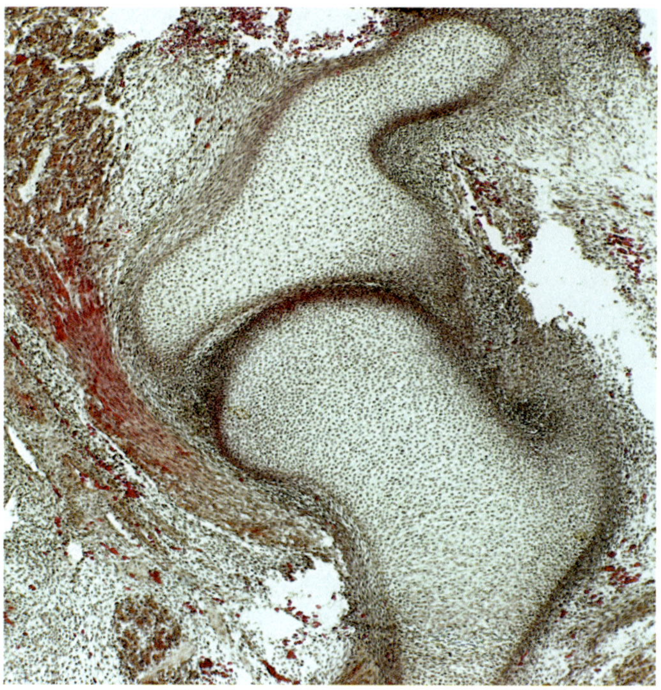

Fig. 12-4. Sagittal section of the hip joint in a 25 mm embryo, showing the beginning of cavitation at the periphery of the interzone. The superior labrum and early capsule are noted. The femoral nerve is clearly visible.

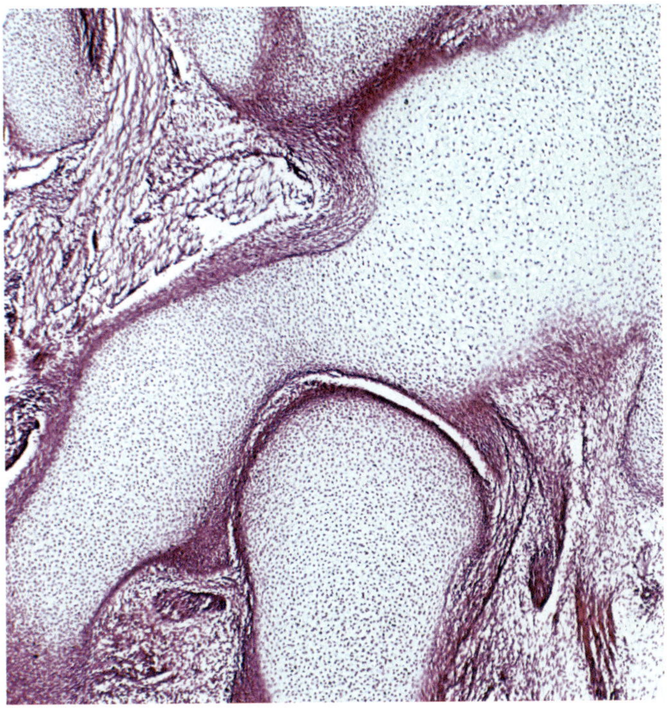

Fig. 12-5. Sagittal section of the hip joint from a 30 mm fetus, showing the sharply defined acetabular labrum. The cavity is well developed. The superior and inferior labra, and joint capsule are seen.

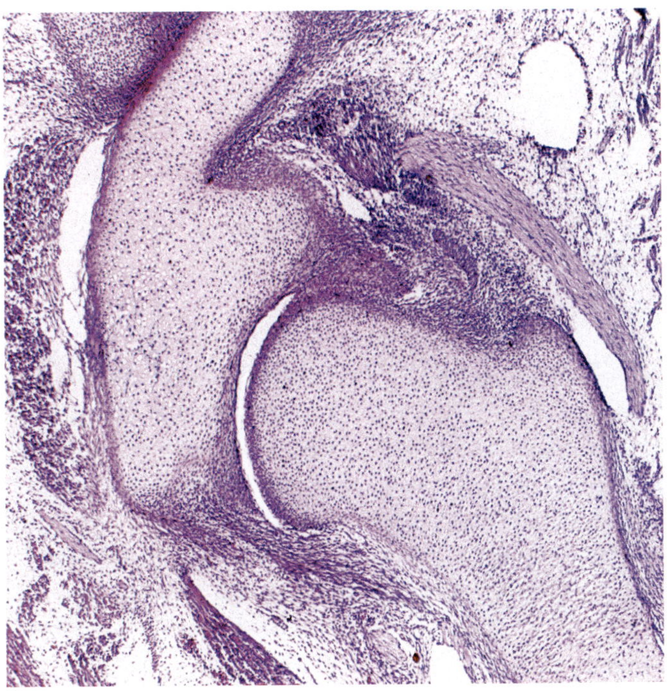

Fig. 12-6. Sagittal section through part of the hip joint in a 35 mm fetus to show the cavity around the head of the femur. The superior labrum and joint capsule are well-formed. The sciatic nerve is well defined.

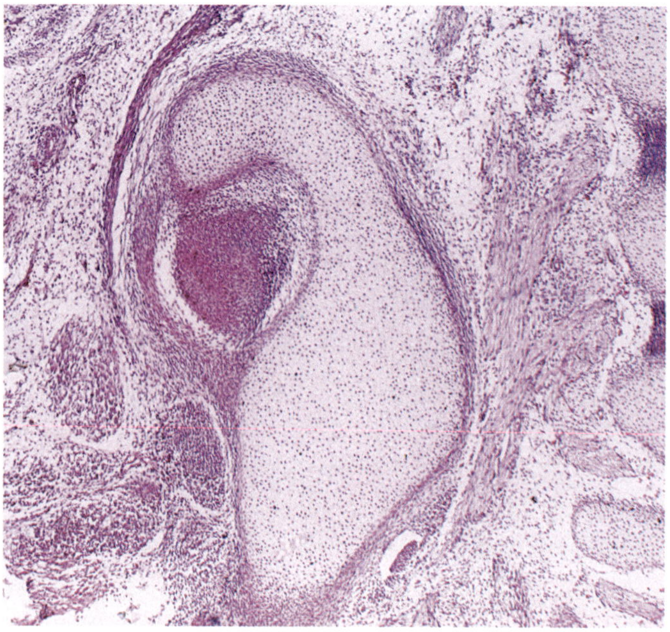

Fig. 12-7. Sagittal section through part of the hip joint from a 35 mm fetus to show the ligament of the head of the femur and transverse acetabular ligament. The iliopsoas muscles and sciatic nerve are seen. The bursa for the tendon of the obturator internus muscle is observed.

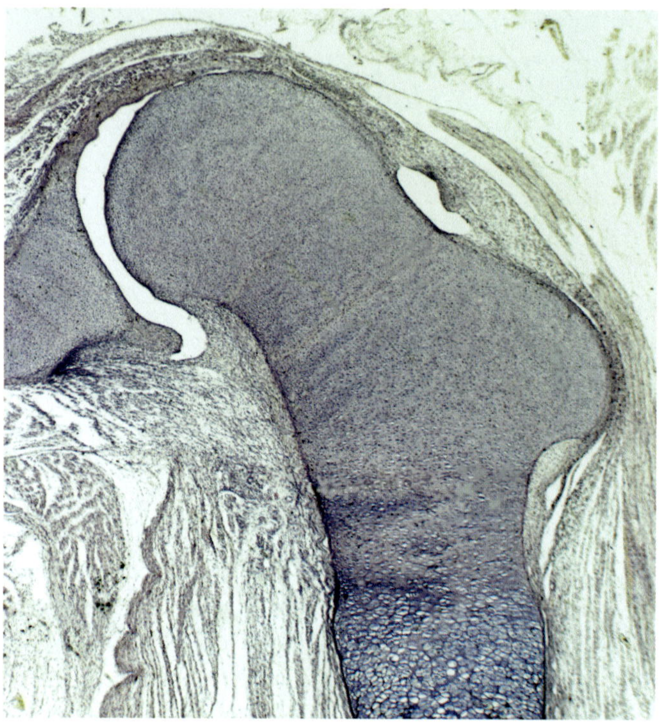

Fig. 12-8. Sagittal section through part of of the hip joint from a 40 mm fetus, showing sharply defined acetabular labrum, cavity, and joint capsule. The thicker part of the capsule indicates zona orbicularis. Early diaphyseal ossification is evident.

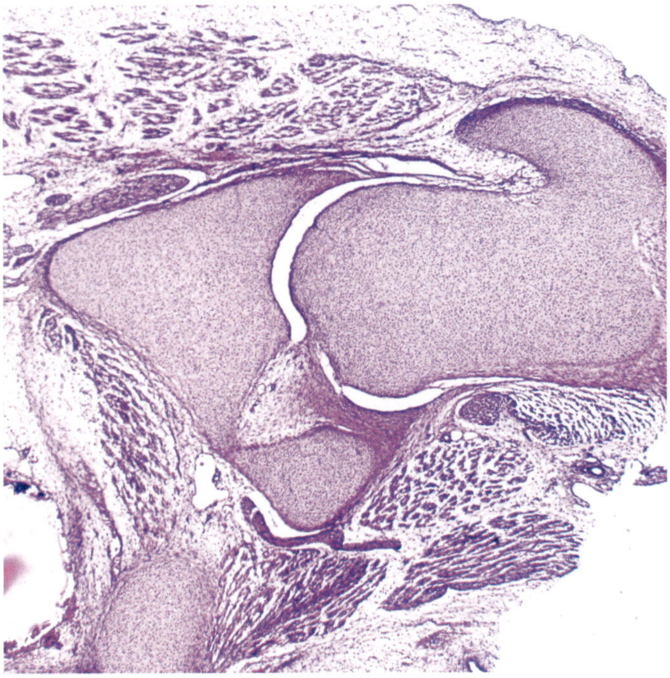

Fig. 12-9. Transverse section through the midportion of the hip joint from a 40 mm fetus, showing acetabular labrum, cavity, and joint capsule. The ligament of head of femur and acetabular fossa are well defined.

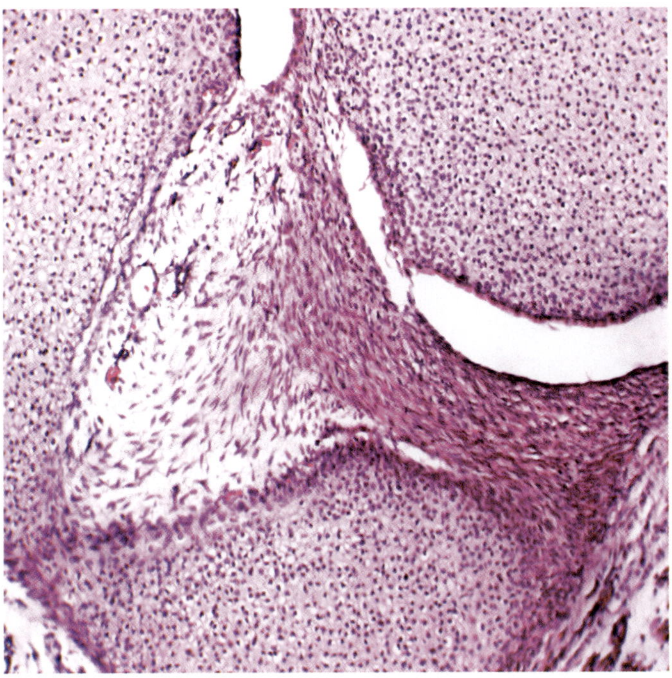

Fig. 12-10. Part of Fig. 12-9 to show the ligament of head of femur. The acetabular fossa is filled with vascular synovial tissue. The ligament of head of femur is composed of densely cellular tissue.

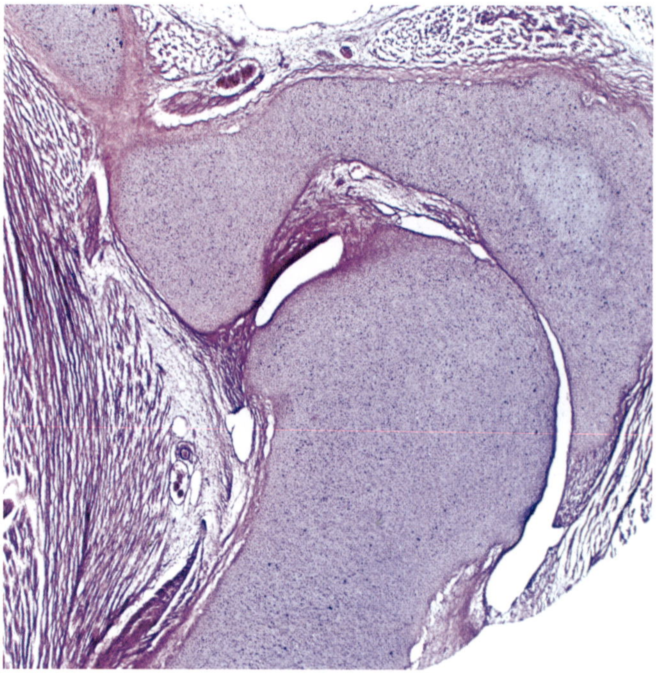

Fig. 12-11. Sagittal section through the medial part of the hip joint from a 55 mm fetus, showing the cavity around the head of femur. The ligament of head of femur, transverse acetabular ligament, fovea capitis femoris, and acetabular fossa are clearly visible. Note the early vascularization at the femoral neck.

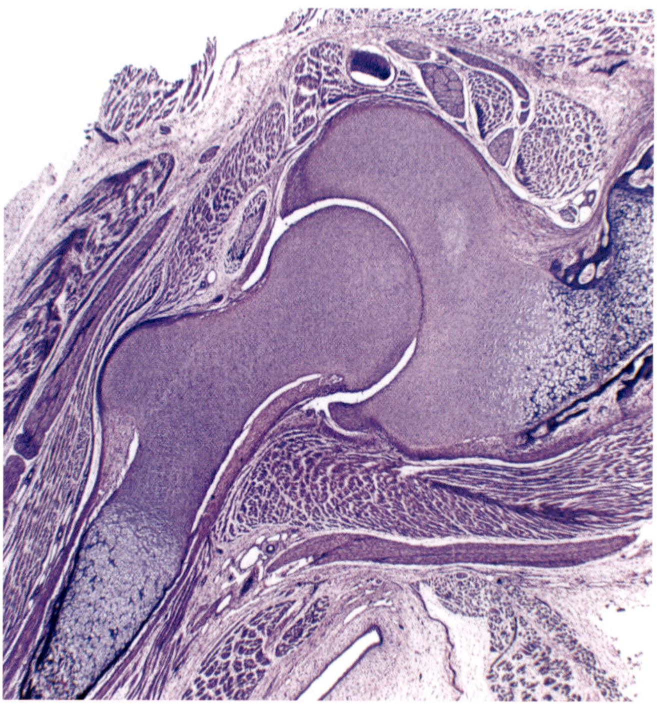

Fig. 12-12. Sagittal section through part of the hip joint from a 60 mm fetus to show the acetabular labrum and zona orbicularis. Endochondral ossification and subperiosteal bone formation of the ilium are seen. The sciatic nerve lies behind the external rotator muscles. The femoral nerve is also seen.

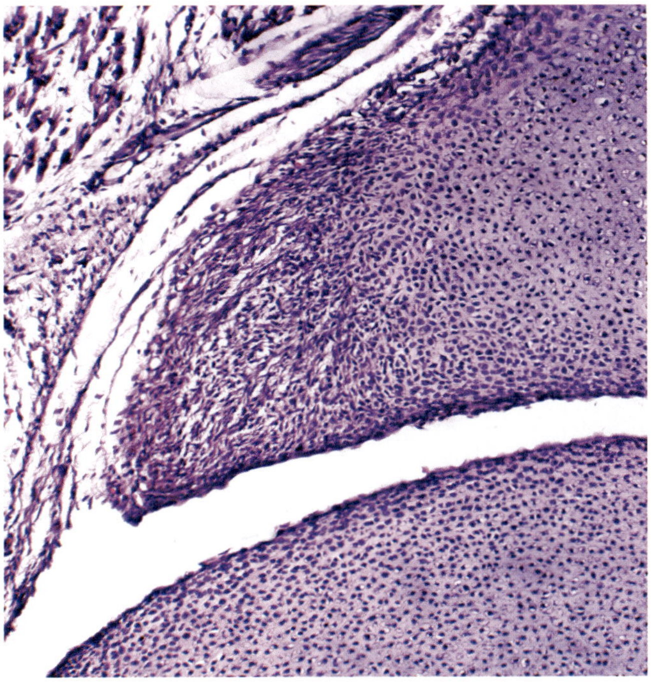

Fig. 12-13. Sagittal section through part of the hip joint in a 60 mm fetus to show the acetabular labrum. The labrum is composed of numerous collagenous bundles and cells, and is clearly demarcated from the adjacent hyaline cartilage.

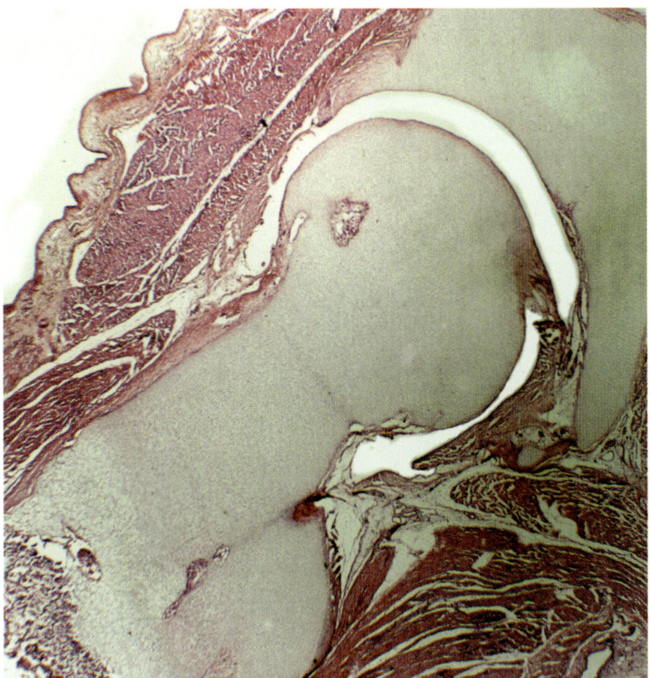

Fig. 12-14. Sagittal section through the midportion of the hip joint from a 70 mm fetus to show cartilage canals in the head of femur. Note the acetabular fossa, fovea capitis femoris, and early vascularization at the femoral neck and near the acetabular labrum. Blood vessels are also seen in the ligament of head of femur.

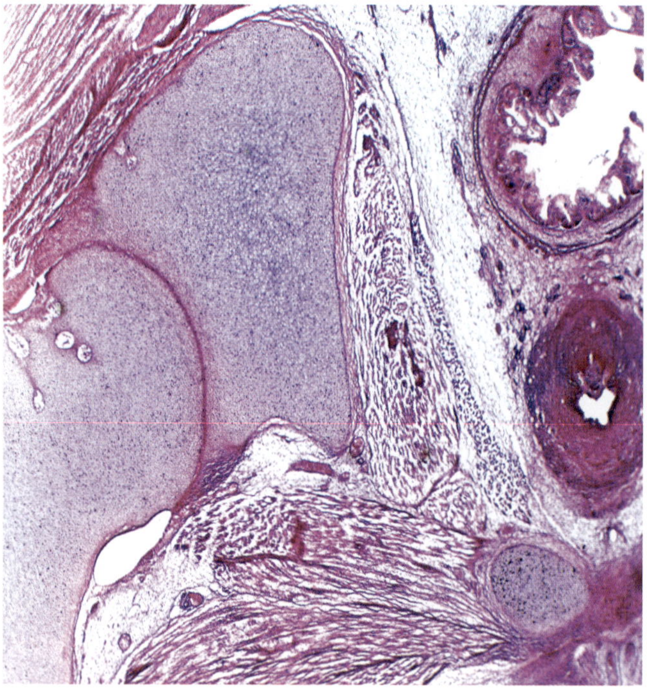

Fig. 12-15. Transverse section through the midportion of the hip joint in a 90 mm fetus, showing the acetabular labrum and joint capsule. Cartilage canals appear in the femoral neck and near the acetabulum.

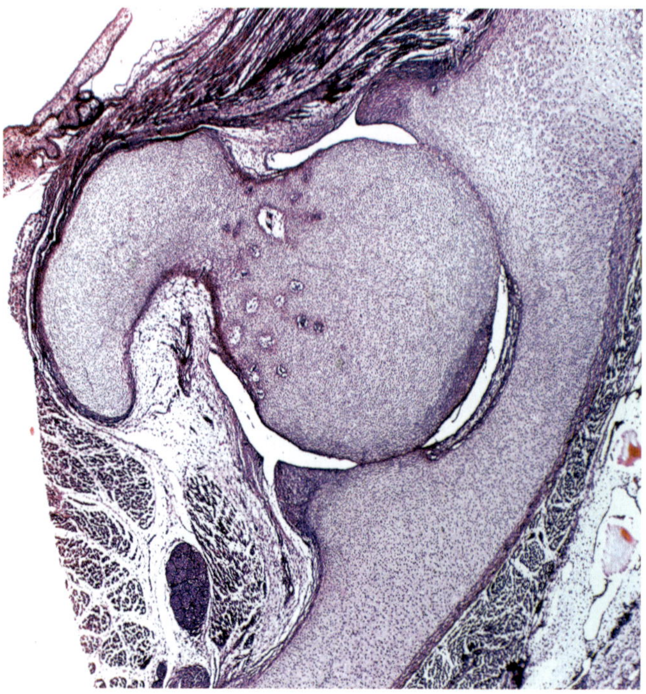

Fig. 12-16. Transverse section through the midportion of the hip joint from a 100 mm fetus to show the acetabular labrum and joint capsule. Cartilage canals in the femoral neck are numerous. The gluteus medius inserts into the perichondrium of the greater trochanter. The sciatic nerve lies behind the external rotator muscles.

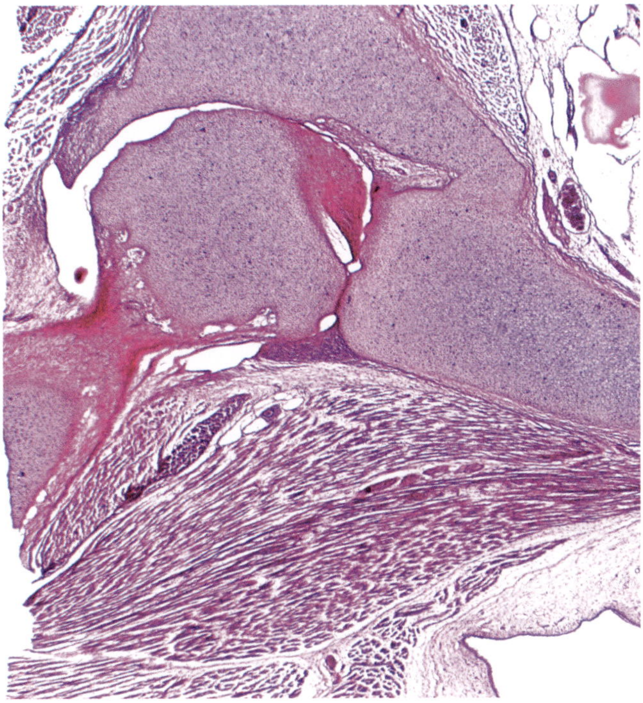

Fig. 12-17. Tranverse section through part of the hip joint from a 110 mm fetus to show the ligament of head of femur and acetabular labrum. Synovial villi are present at the angle of reflection of the synovial tissue and synovial folds passed from the acetabular fossa to the margin of the fovea capitis femoris.

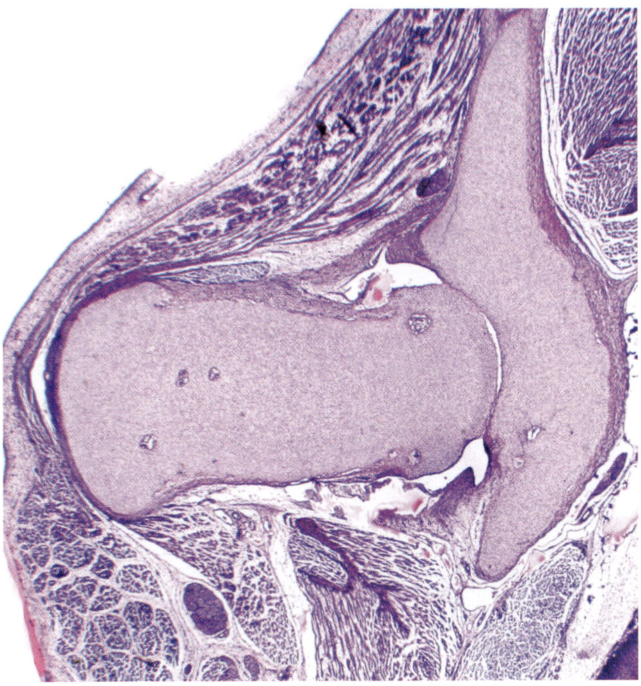

Fig. 12-18. Transverse section through the midportion of the hip joint in a 130 mm fetus to show the acetabular labrum and joint capsule. Cartilage canals appear in the femoral head and acetabulum. The gluteus medius inserts into the perichondrium of the greater trochanter.

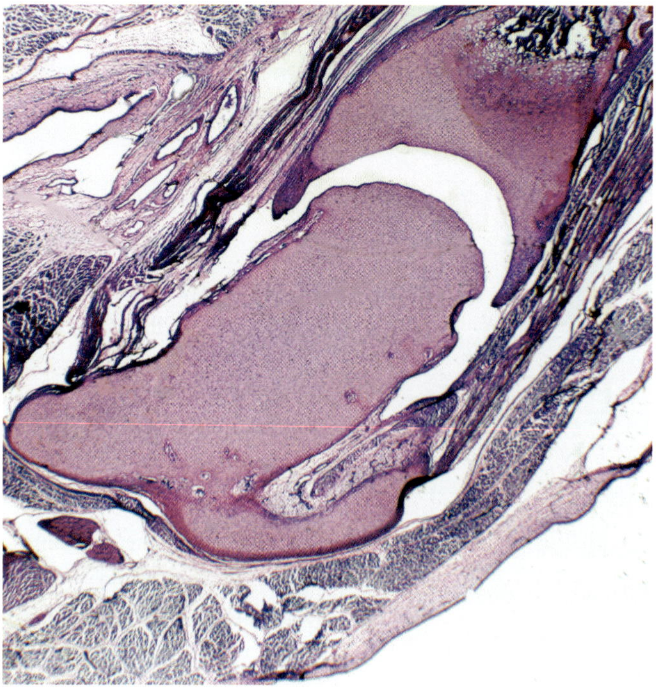

Fig. 12-19. Transverse section of the hip joint from a 130 mm fetus to show increased ossification and vascularization. Ossification of the ilium approaches the acetabulum. Note the longitudinal section of the arteriole as well as the cross section of venule of the synovial tissue.

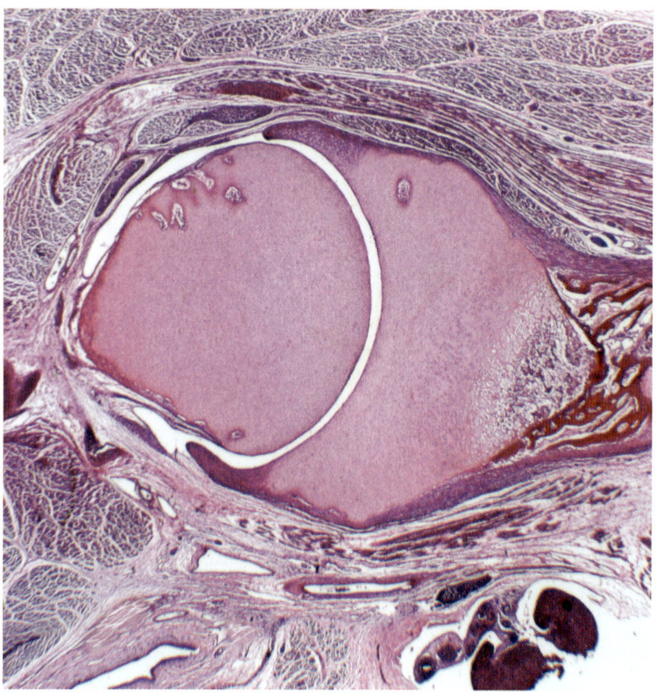

Fig. 12-20. Transverse section through the midportion of the hip joint in a 160 mm fetus, showing advancing ossification and vascularization. Vascularization is considerably advanced and ligaments are well defined. The sciatic nerve is clearly visible. The endochondral ossification and periosteal bone formation of the ilium are seen.

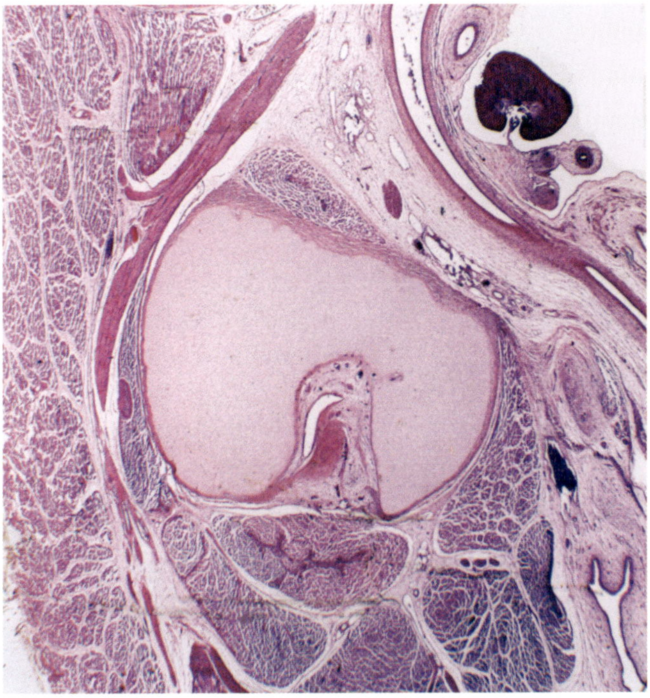

Fig. 12-21. Transverse section of the hip joint from a 160 mm fetus, showing the acetabular fossa and transverse acetabular ligament. Note the part of a synovial fold near the acetabular fossa containing small blood vessels. The sciatic nerve is clearly visible. Adipose tissue is present as isolated cells in the acetabular fossa.

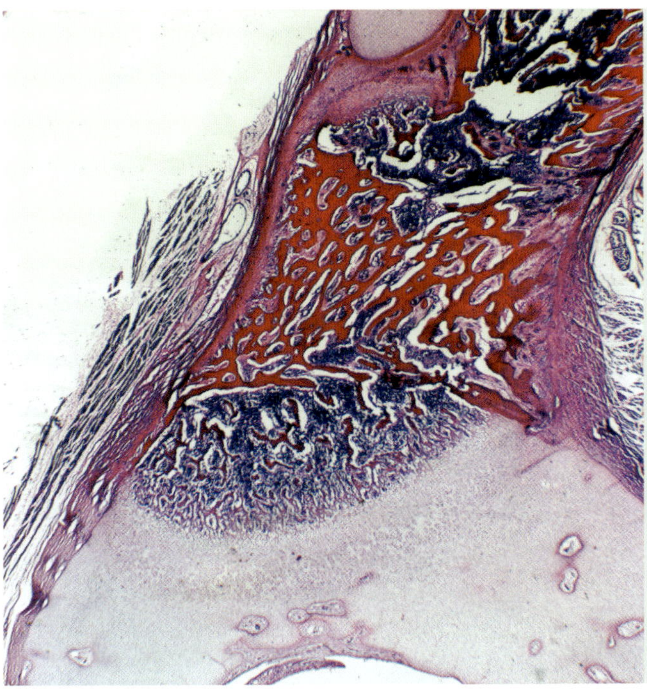

Fig. 12-22. Sagittal section through the midportion of the acetabulum from a 230 mm fetus showing the extent of the endochondral ossification in the ilium. The center of ossification extends laterally and inferiorly into the base of the acetabular limbus. Cartilage canals are numerous in the acetabulum.

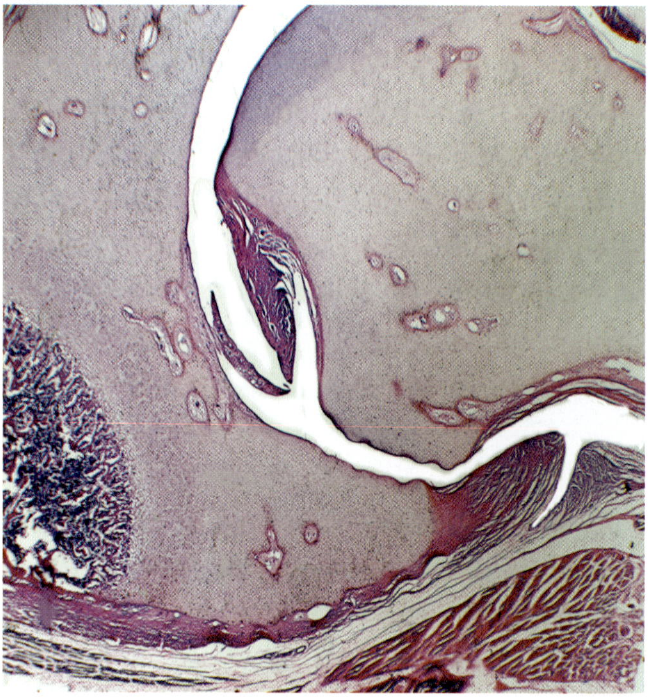

Fig. 12-23. Sagittal section through the midportion of the hip joint from a 230 mm fetus, showing the fibrous acetabular labrum. The ossification of the ilium is approaching the acetabulum. Cartilage canals in the femoral head and acetabulum are seen. Note the rich vascularization of the acetabular fossa.

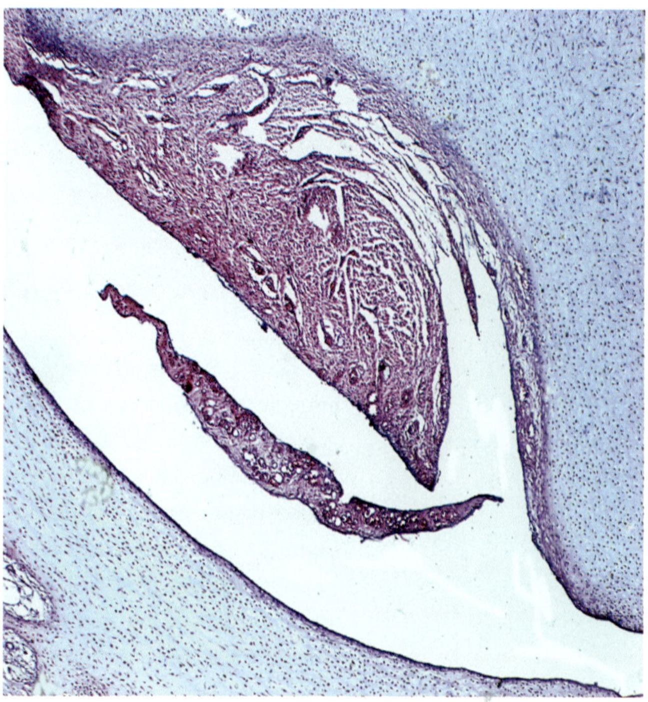

Fig. 12-24. Part of Fig. 12-23 to show the rich vascularization of the ligament of head of femur. The fovea capitis femoris is filled with a vascular tissue which is sharply demarcated from articular cartilage.

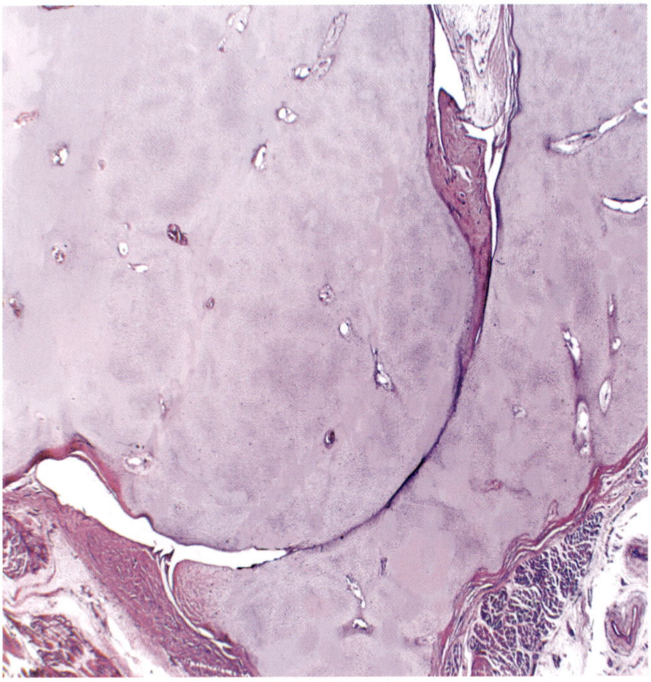

Fig. 12-25. Frontal section through part of hip joint from a 260 mm fetus to show the ligament of head of femur and fovea capitis femoris. Cartilage canals are numerous in the femoral head and acetabulum.

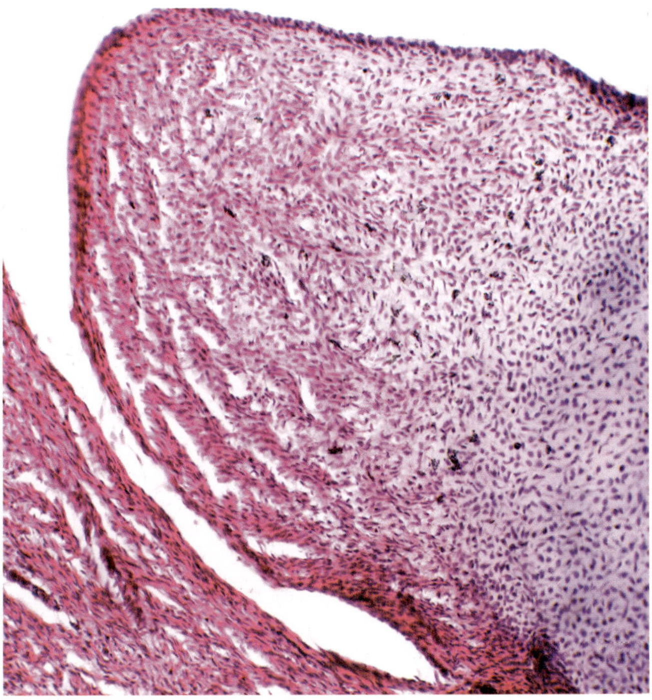

Fig. 12-26. Part of Fig. 12-25 to show the sharply defined acetabular labrum. The labrum is composed of numerous collagenous bundles and fibroblasts and is clearly demarcated from the adjacent hyaline cartilage.

References

Bardeen CR, Lewis WH: Development of the limb, body-wall and back in man. *Am J Anat* 1: 1-45, 1901.

DeSanto DA, Colonna PC: Embryology of the hip joint. *Arch Surg* 39: 448-456, 1939.

Gardner E, Gray DJ: Prenatal development of the human hip joint. *Am J Anat* 87: 163-211, 1950.

Kim KL: The prenatal development of the hip joint in Korean fetus. *Chonnam Medical J* 6: 343-362, 1969.

The Development of the Knee Joint

Chapter 13

The primordium of the femur, the tibia and the knee joint can be recognized to appear as skeletal blastema from the 15 mm embryo (Fig. 13-1), and to complete the chondrification in the 27 mm embryo (Fig. 13-4). The patella, formed in the 22 mm embryo as the cellular differentiation of the quadriceps femoris tendon (Fig. 13-3), is observed to finish the chondrification in the 40 mm fetus (Figs. 13-6).

Cartilage canals are present in the proximal tibial epiphysis in 50 mm fetus (Fig. 13-12). By the 70 mm fetus, cartilage canals are observed to contain a number of thin-walled blood vessels, and loose connective tissue (Fig. 13-19). The vessels originated from perichondral vascular network at regular intervals and some of them communicated with those in the diaphysis. In the 90 mm fetus, cartilage canals of the distal femur, proximal tibia, and patella are first seen (Fig. 13-20). At this stage, endochondral ossification of the femur and tibia reaches the metaphyseal areas. As endochondral ossification of the femur and tibia extends proximally and distally, growth zones become established in the 200 mm fetus (Figs. 13-28). After the 260 mm fetus, the extent of endochondral and perichondral ossification are the same (Fig. 13-30).

The homogenous interzone and three-layered interzone in the knee joint are present in the 15 mm and 20 mm embryos (Figs. 13-1 and 13-2). The knee joint is noted to assume the form of a normal joint surface from the 22 mm embryo, and its intermediate layer proceeds developing as the vascular mesenchymal cells which are closely incorporated with the periarticular chondrogenous layer (Fig. 13-5). By the 30 mm fetus, the primitive joint space is first seen in the three-layered interzone as a narrow cleft around the periphery (Fig. 13-6). No degenerative phenomena of the intermediate layer of the interzone are noticed. Recognition of the femoropatellar joint, both femoromeniscal and tibiomeniscal joints, is possible in the 22 mm (Fig. 13-3) and 27 mm embryos, respectively (Fig. 13-5). Primitive joint cavities of all these joints are observed for the first time in the 35 mm fetus (Fig. 13-7).

Development of the patellar ligament begins to form as a continuation of the developing quadriceps muscle in the 22 mm embryo (Fig. 13-3). The intra-articular structures develop in situ from the intermediate layer of the interzone. By the 27 mm embryo, the appearance of the primordium of the cruciate ligament and the meniscus is conspicuous as the vascular mesenchymal cells, proceeding to that of joint space (Figs. 13-4 and 13-5). The collateral ligaments begin to form as a condensation of the joint capsule in the 27 mm embryo (Fig. 13-5).

By the 60 mm fetus, the cells in the menisci have increased in size and the collagenous fibers are more prominent (Figs. 13-17 and 13-18). In the 105 mm fetus, the menisci are composed of loosely arranged fibroblasts which appear to be more voluminous in the inner zones, and smaller and more compactly arranged in the middle and outer zones (Fig. 13-22). During the next prenatal stage up to the 170 mm fetus, the inner zone of the meniscus is filled with parallelly oriented fascicles of collagenous fibers and oval fibroblasts. The middle zone of the meniscus consists of radially arranged fibroblasts and chondroid cells. The outer zone of the meniscus is populated by elongated fibroblasts encircled by intercrossed collagenous fibers with the blood vessels (Fig. 13-26).

The individual cavities enlarge, coalesce, and form a single cavity in the 40 mm fetus (Fig. 13-8). Synovial villi are first noted in the suprapatellar pouch in the 55 mm fetus (Fig. 13-13). The vascularity of the synovial tissue has increased, and synovial villi are present in the infrapatellar region in the 130 and 170 mm fetuses (Figs. 13-24 and 13-25). The synovial folds contain numerous bundles of collagenous fiber as well as central arterioles and venules in the 250 mm fetus (Fig. 13-29). By the 130 mm fetus, several different types of cells are seen in the synovial membrane (Fig. 13-24).

By the 30 mm fetus, scattered fat cells are first noted in the infrapatellar region (Fig. 13-9). Development of the infrapatellar fat pad is evident in the 50 mm fetus (Fig. 13-11). The infrapatellar fold is markedly vascular, especially near the joint cavity in the 90 mm fetus (Fig. 13-20). In the 200 mm fetus, the lobules of fat are large, fat cells found along the cruciate ligaments (Figs. 13-27 and 13-29).

By the 40 mm fetus, the tendon of the popliteus is separated from the lateral meniscus posterolaterally by a synovial recess of the joint cavity (Fig. 13-10). Fabella is present in the lateral head of the gastrocnemius of the 105 mm fetus (Fig. 13-21).

The superior tibiofibular joint cavity is first noted in the 40 mm fetus and a connection between this cavity and the lateral tibiomeniscal cavity is visible (Fig. 13-10). In most cases, the cavity of the knee joint is separated from that of the superior tibiofibullar joint by a small amount of loose connective tissue (Fig. 13-14).

The first morphological evidence of secondary center of ossification in the distal femoral chondroepiphysis is found in the 300 mm fetus (Fig. 13-30). At one month of age, with the progressive development of the secondary ossification center, the epiphyseal plate becomes well differentiated and shows a typical zonal differentiation (Fig. 13-31). Once the bony center appears, ossification along the articular side of the secondary center is different from that along the metaphyseal side. As the secondary center expands toward the metaphysis, many cartilage cells bordering the metaphyseal side of the secondary center do not degenerate (Fig. 13-32).

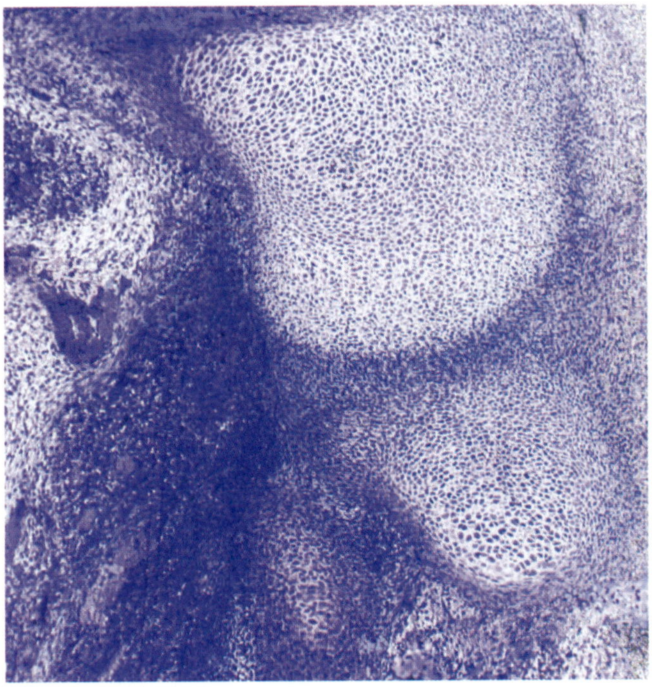

Fig. 13-1. Frontal section through the knee joint from a 15 mm embryo to show chondrification of the femur, tibia, and fibulla. Homogenous interzone in the knee joint is seen.

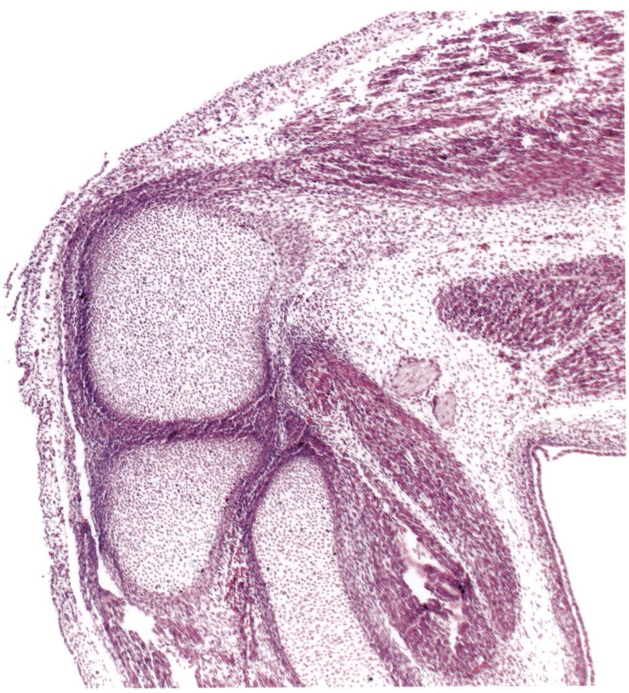

Fig. 13-2. Sagittal section through the knee joint from a 20 mm embryo to show chondrification of the femur, tibia, and fibula. The three-layered interzone is located between the femur and tibia. The three-layered interzone of the superior tibiofibular joint is also seen. The common peroneal nerve passes through the gastrocnemius.

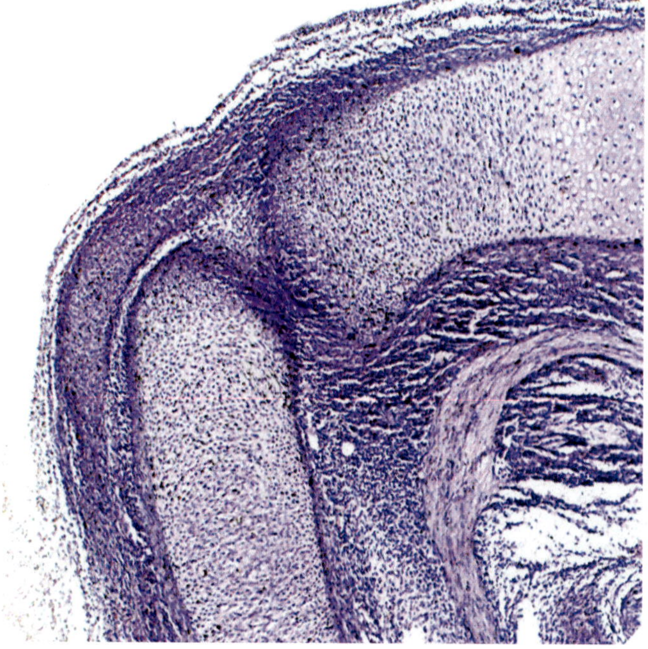

Fig. 13-3. Sagittal section through the knee joint from a 22 mm embryo to show a three-layered interzone. The quadriceps tendon, hamstring muscles, patellar tendon, and sciatic nerve are clearly visible. The organization of the patellofemoral cavity has begun.

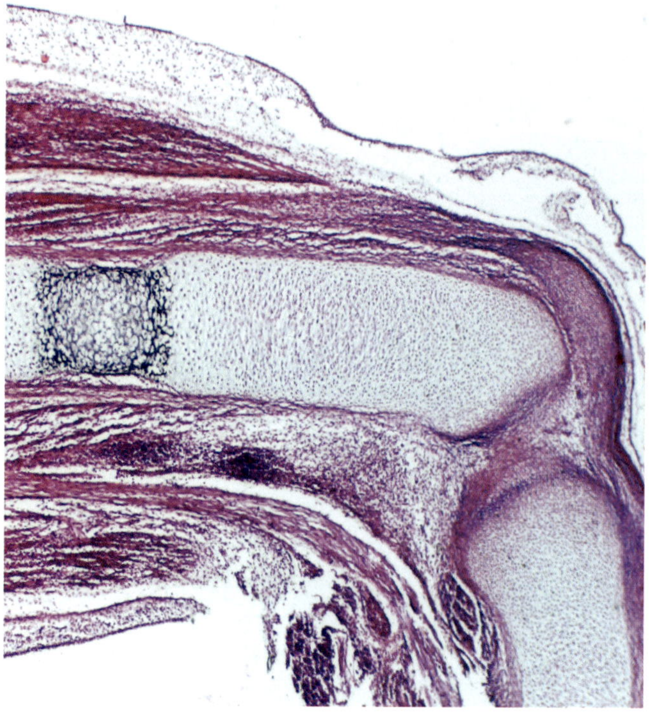

Fig. 13-4. Sagittal section through the knee joint from a 27 mm embryo to show condensation for anterior and posterior cruciate ligaments. The quadriceps tendon and patellar ligament are seen. Note the extent of the ossification in the shaft of the femur.

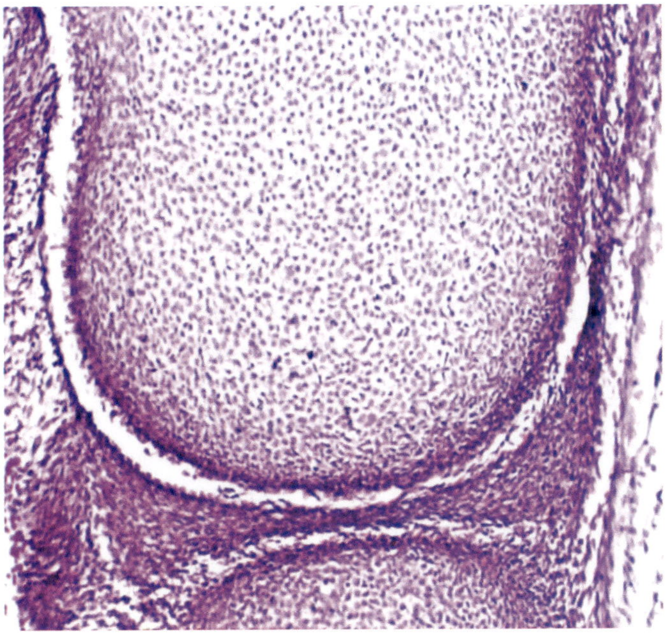

Fig. 13-5. Sagittal section through the knee joint from a 27 mm embryo to show the medial meniscus. Formation of the femoromeniscal and tibiomeniscal joint cavities has begun. Both cavities are crossed by conjunctive mesenchymal tissue. The joint capsules are attached to the peripheral margin of the menisci.

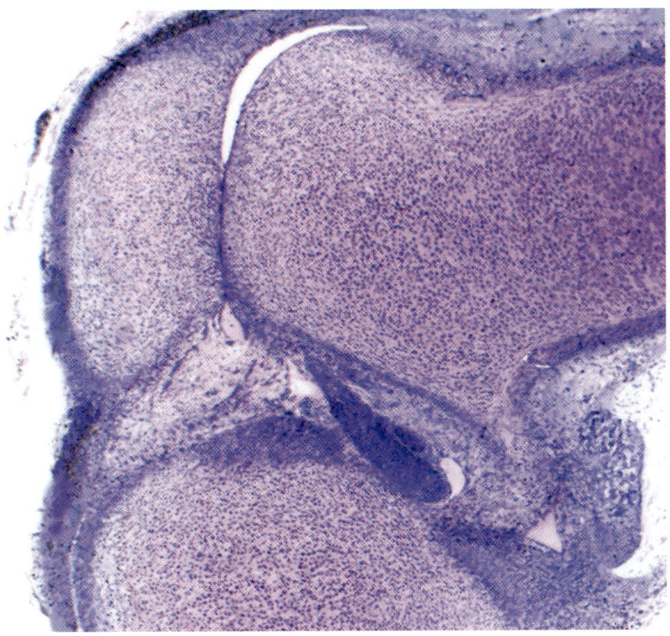

Fig. 13-6. Sagittal section of the knee joint from a 30 mm fetus to show peripheral cavitation between the femur and patella. Anterior and posterior cruciate ligaments are seen. A triangular space forms in the infrapatellar region. This space is occupied by mesenchymal tissue.

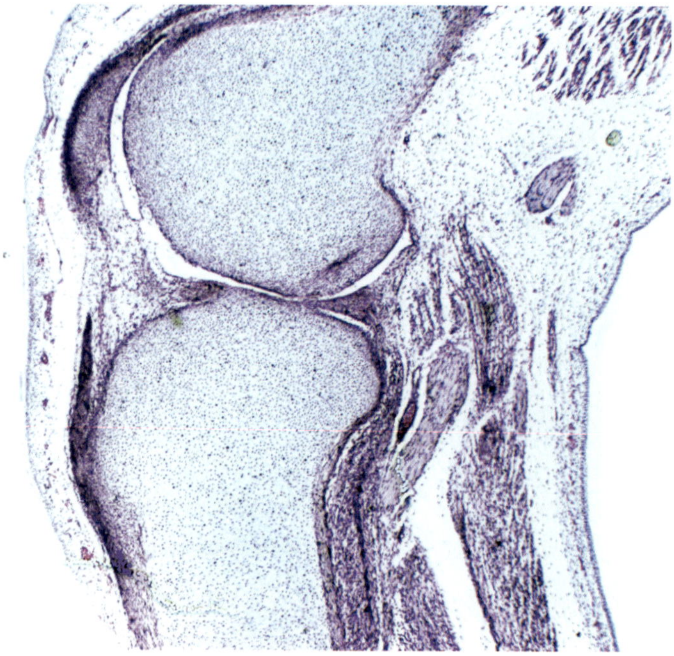

Fig. 13-7. Sagittal section through the knee joint in the 35 mm fetus, showing femoropatellar, femoromeniscal, and tibiomeniscal joint cavities. The menisci are well defined. Cavities are present superior and inferior to the medial meniscus. The fibrous capsule is poorly developed. The common peroneal nerve and gastrocnemius muscle are seen.

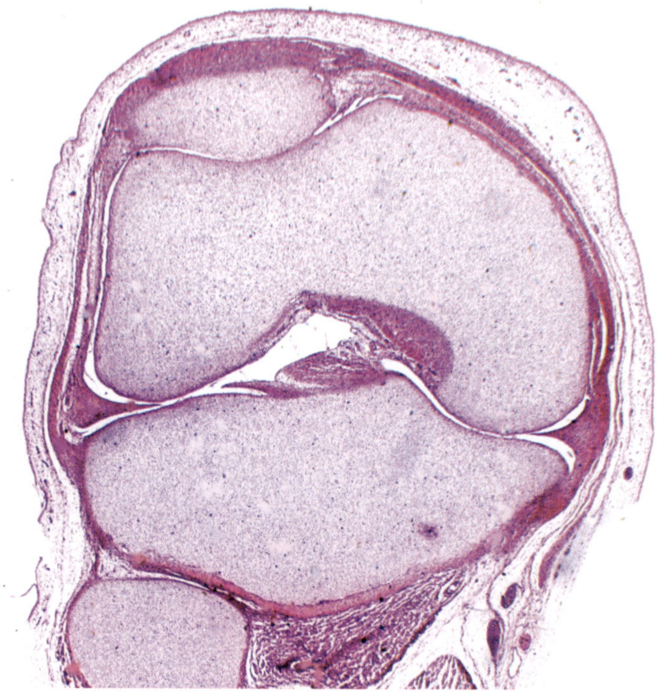

Fig. 13-8. Frontal section through the knee joint from a 40 mm fetus, showing the patellar retinacula. The joint cavities are present superior and inferior to the both menisci. Anterior cruciate ligament and menisci are clearly visible. Development of the collateral ligaments begin as a condensation of the joint capsule.

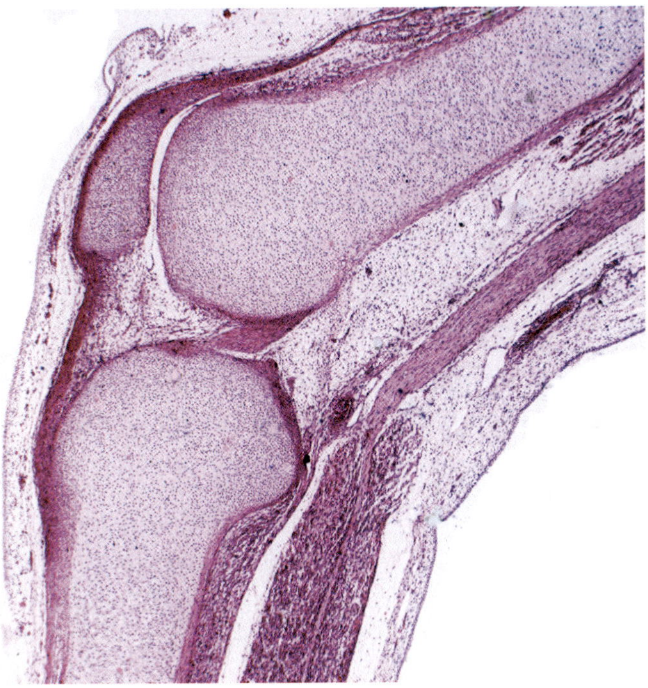

Fig. 13-9. Sagittal section through the knee joint from a 40 mm fetus, showing the patellofemoral joint. The quadriceps tendon and the patellar and anterior cruciate ligaments are seen. The infrapatellar fat pad begins to form. This fat pad is located between the anterior cruciate and patellar ligaments. The sciatic and common peroneal nerves are clearly visible.

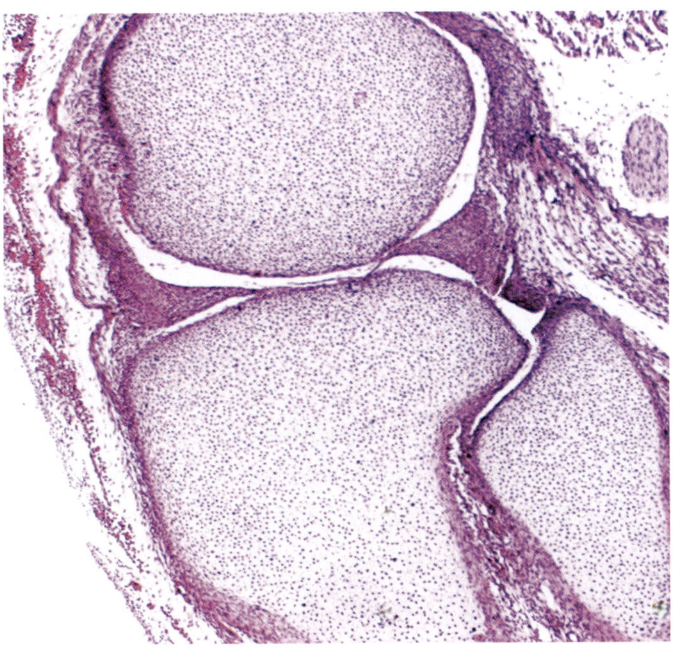

Fig. 13-10. Frontal section through the knee joint in a 40 mm fetus to show the superior tibiofibular joint. The cavity of the knee joint communicates with that of the superior tibiofibular joint. The tendon of the popliteus muscle is separated from the lateral meniscus. The medial and lateral menisci are completely formed, and femoromeniscal and tibiomeniscal joint cavities are established.

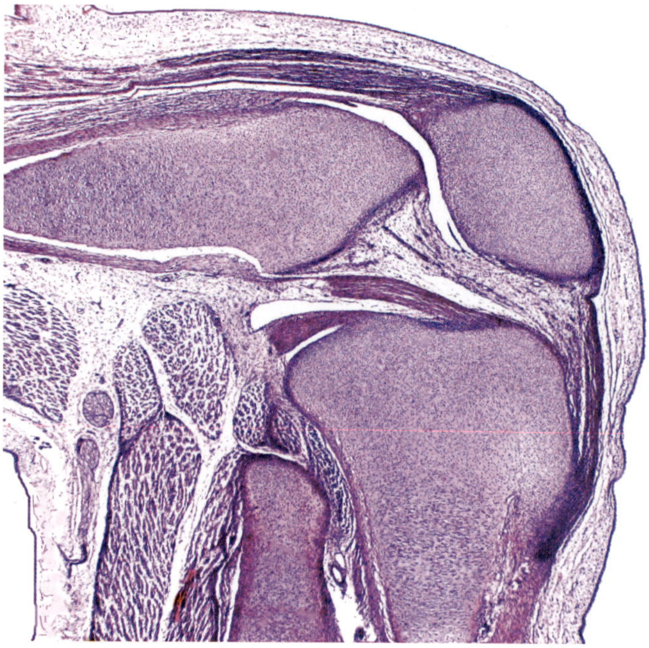

Fig. 13-11. Sagittal section through the knee joint from a 50 mm fetus, showing the extent of the cavity and also in relation to the menisci. The degree of developmemt of the infrapatellar fat pad is evident. This fat pad is attached to the intercondylar fossa of the femur. A small cavity is located behind the anterior cruciate ligament.

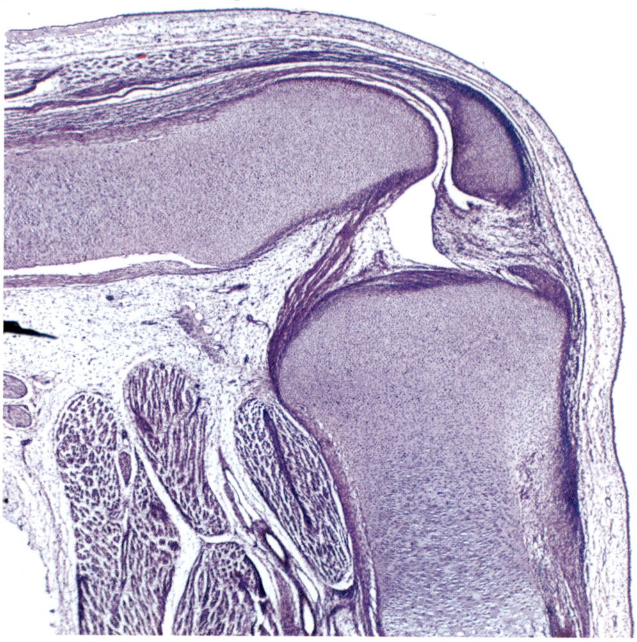

Fig. 13-12. Sagittal section through the knee joint from a 50 mm fetus, showing villus projecting into the cavity from the synovial membrane. A joint cavity is located anterior to the posterior cruciate ligament. Vascularization of the tibial epiphysis is just beginning as cartilage canals enter the tibia, the regions near the tuberosity of the tibia, and near the posterior condyle.

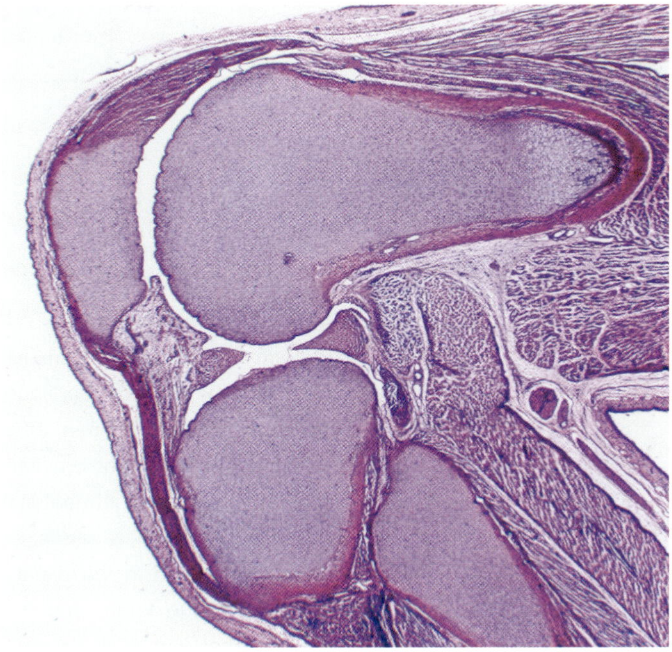

Fig. 13-13. Sagittal section of the knee joint from a 55 mm fetus to show extensive joint cavitation, meniscus, and synovial membrane. The synovial tissue is loose and vascular. Small folds and villi are found. The initial appearance of the cartilage canals in the femur is seen.

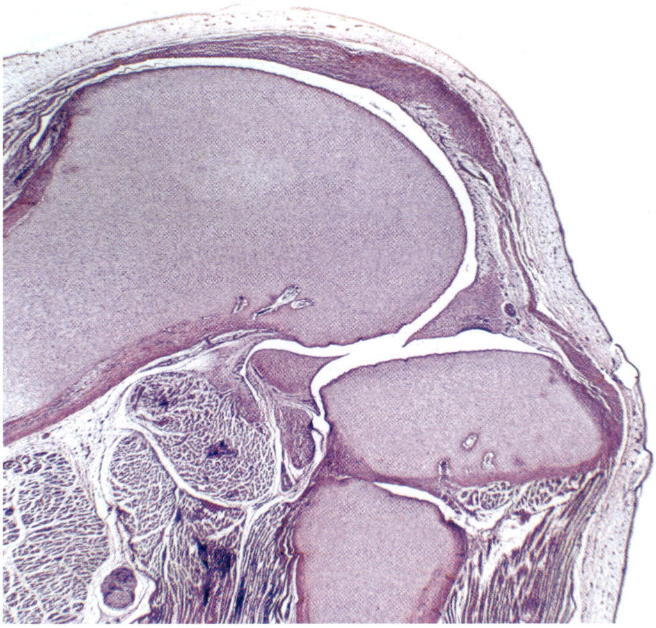

Fig. 13-14. Sagittal section of the knee joint from a 60 mm fetus to show cartilage canals in the distal femur and proximal tibia. The cavity of the knee joint is separated from that of the superior tibiofibular joint by a small amount of loose tissue.

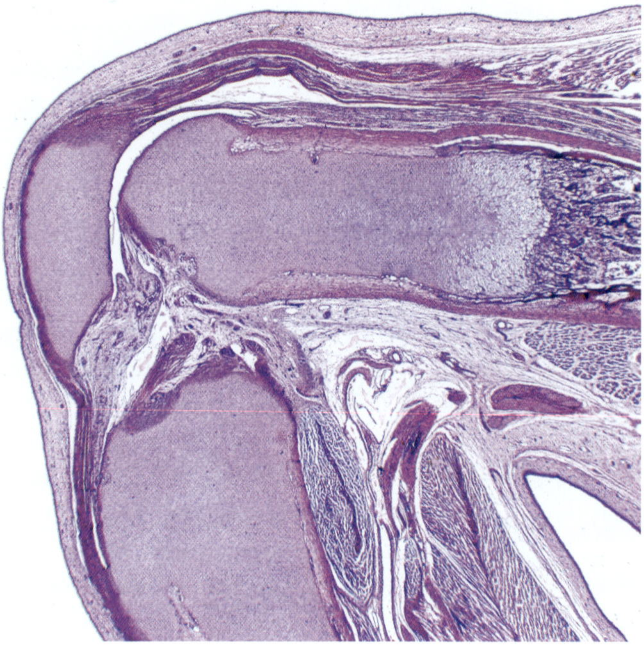

Fig. 13-15. Sagittal section through the knee joint from a 60 mm fetus to show cartilage canals in the distal femur and proximal tibia. Anterior cruciate ligament and loose infrapatellar tissue are seen. The cartilage canals are noted in the distal extremity of the femur and in the proximal end of the tibia.

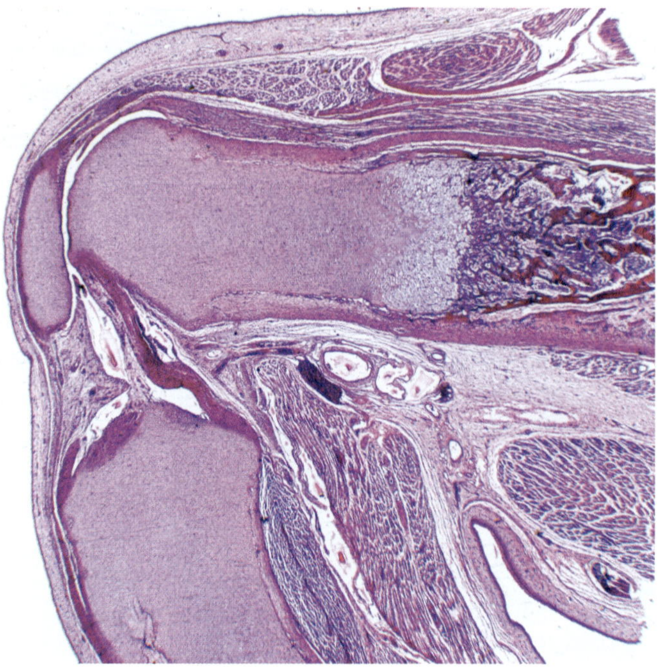

Fig. 13-16. Sagittal section through the knee joint in a 60 mm fetus to show the patellar and posterior cruciate ligaments. Tibial attachment of the posterior cruciate ligament is compact in contrast to the femoral attachment. Small lobules of the fat are present in the infrapatellar region. The beginning of the formation of tibial tuberosity is seen by a vessel invading the proximal epiphysis.

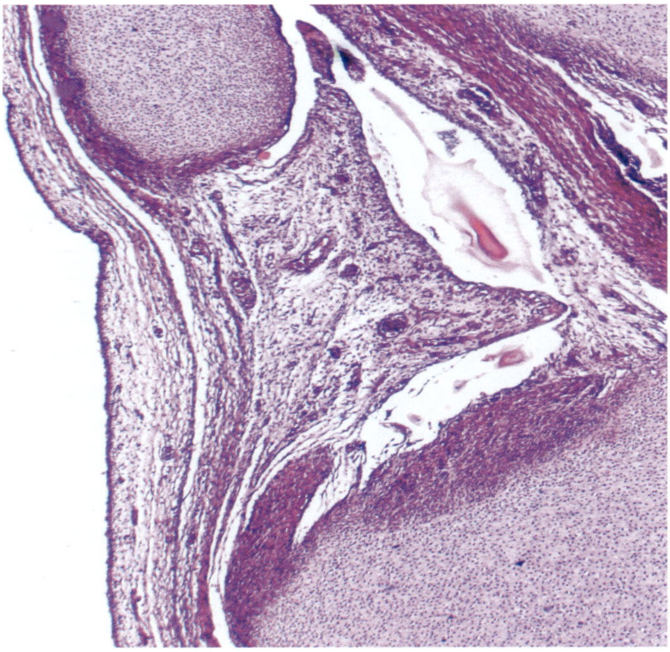

Fig, 13-17. Sagittal section through knee joint from a 60 mm fetus to show the vascular invasion in the synovial mesenchyme. Small folds and villi are found.

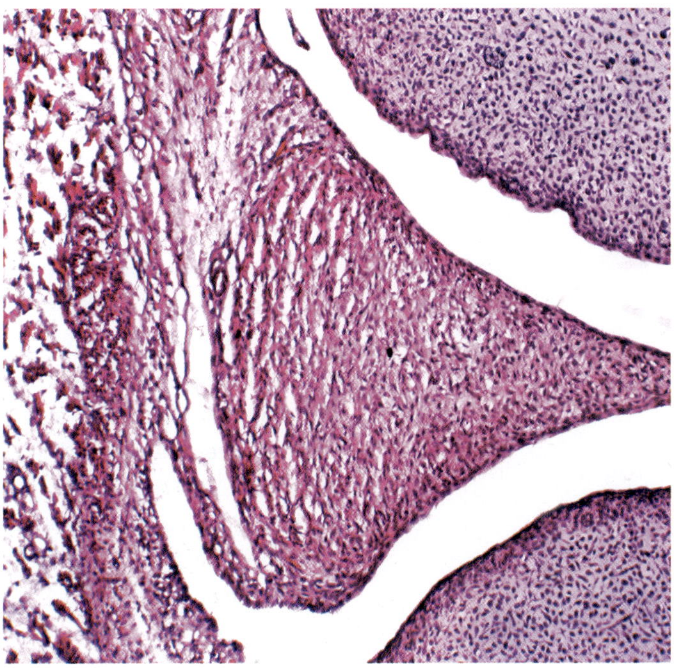

Fig. 13-18. Sagittal section through the knee joint in a 60 mm fetus to show the densely packed fibroblasts of the meniscus. Note the progressive decrease in cellularity and increase in the intercellular matrix with the increasing maturation.

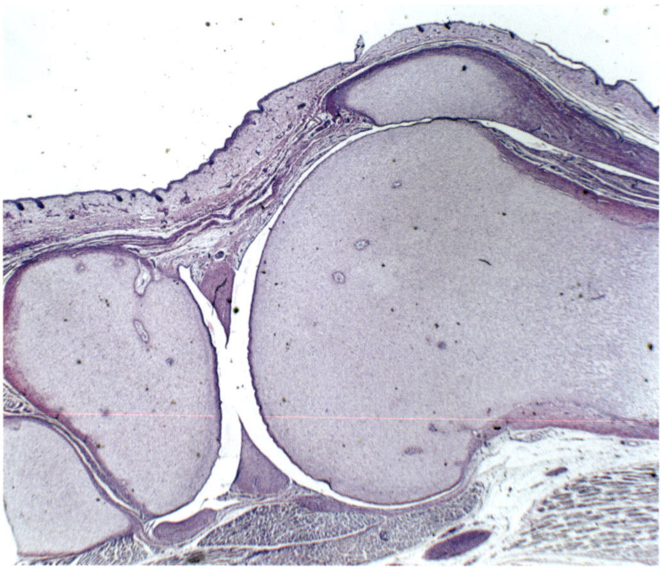

Fig. 13-19. Sagittal section through the knee joint from a 70 mm fetus, showing the lateral meniscus and tendon of the popliteus. Cartilage canals in tibial and femoral condyles are seen. Vessels can be seen entering the tibia from the infrapatellar region.

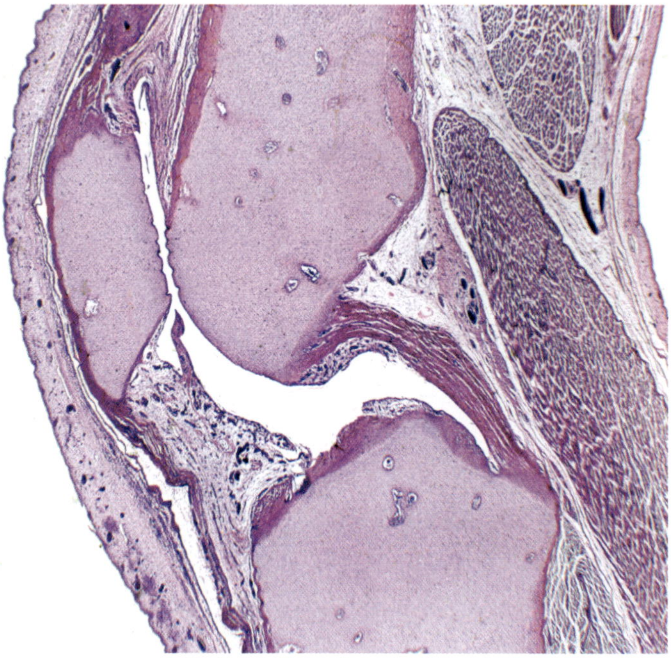

Fig. 13-20. Sagittal section through the knee joint in a 90 mm fetus to show cartilage canals. Cartilage canals can be seen entering the patella from the prepatellar region. A strong posterior cruciate ligament is observed. The infrapatellar fold is markedly vascular, especially near the joint cavity. A plica is noted coming in from the medial side.

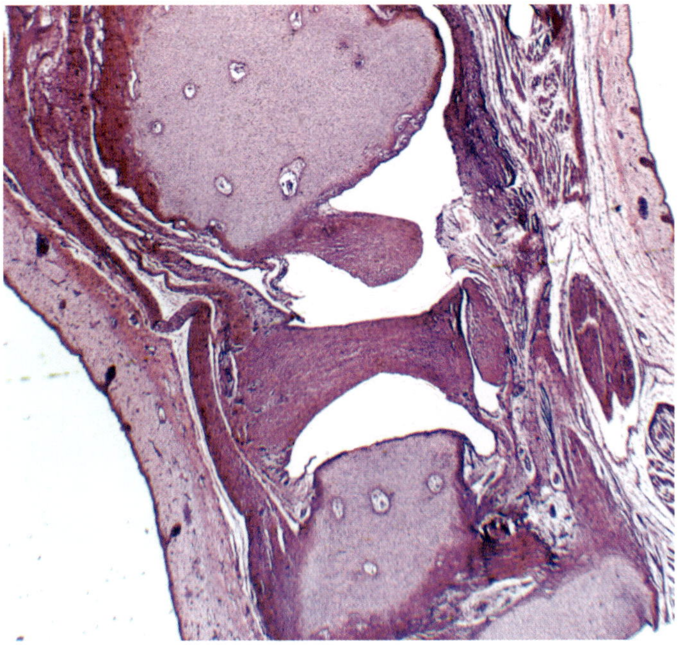

Fig. 13-21. Sagittal section through the knee joint from a 105 mm fetus to show the lateral meniscus. Vessels are seen to enter from the loose tissue to which the meniscus is attached. Cartilage canals in the femur, tibia, and fibula are numerous. Recess of the joint cavity commonly separates the lateral meniscus from the tendon of popliteus muscle. The meniscus is unattached in this region except for the lower margin of its outer aspect.

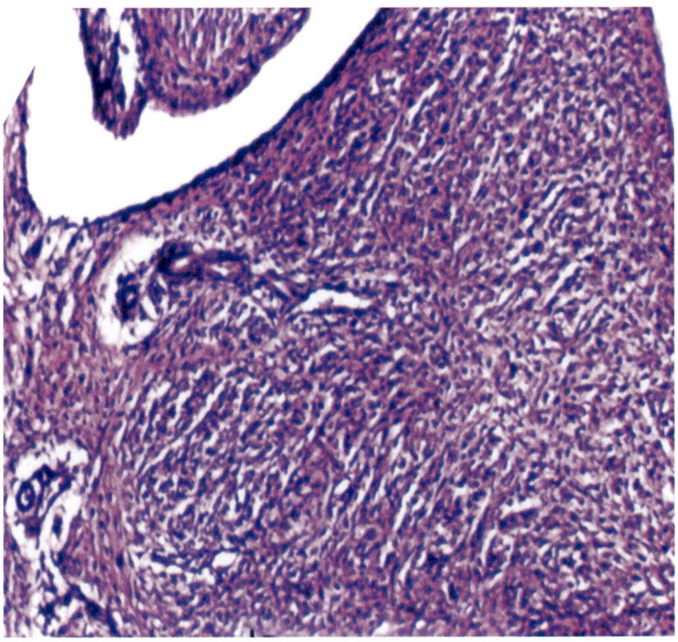

Fig. 13-22. Sagittal section through part of the knee joint from a 105 mm fetus, showing the fibroblasts, collagenous fibers, and blood vessels of the lateral meniscus. Intercrossed collagenous fibers and capillaries are found in the outer zone.

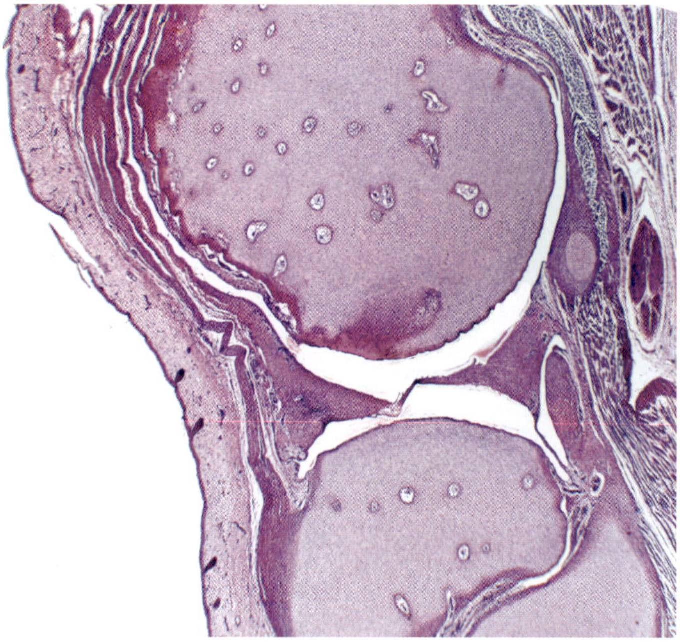

Fig. 13-23. Sagittal section through the knee joint from a 105 mm fetus to show cartilage canals of the distal femur and proximal tibia. A fabella is located in the lateral head of the gastrocnemius muscle. The cavity of the knee joint lies anterior to the fabella.

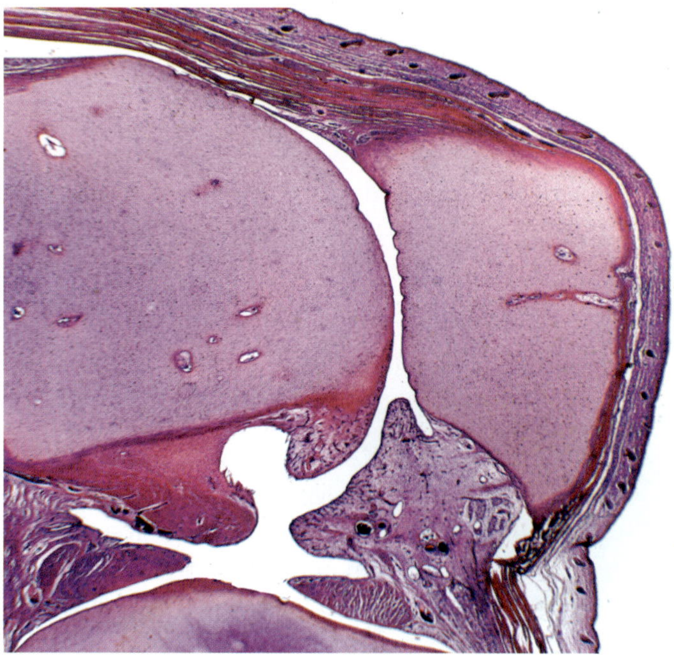

Fig. 13-24. Sagittal section through the part of knee joint from a 130 mm fetus to show the synovial membrane. The cartilage canal penetrates the anterior aspect of the patella. Several villi project into the joint cavity posteriorly.

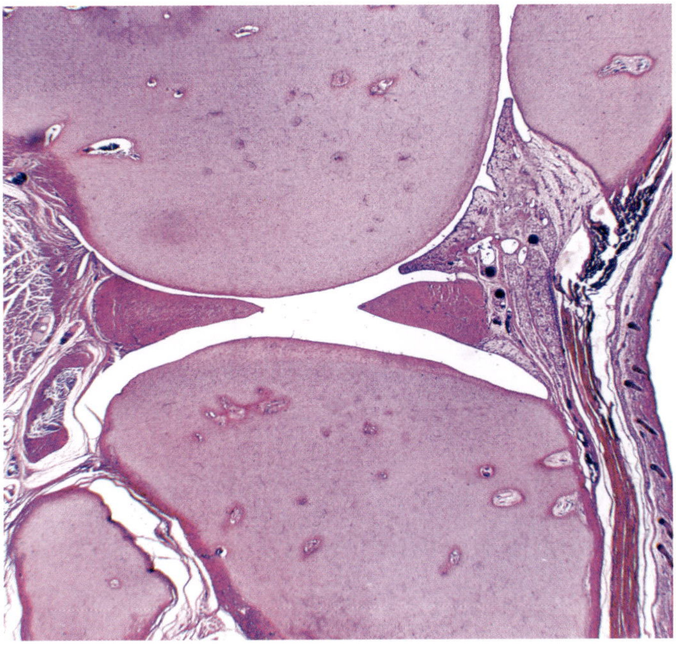

Fig. 13-25. Sagittal section through the knee joint from a 170 mm fetus to show the menisci and synovial tissues. Cartilage canals in the epiphysis of the distal femur, proximal tibia, and fibula are numerous. The communication between the superior tibiofibular and lateral meniscofibular joint cavities is seen.

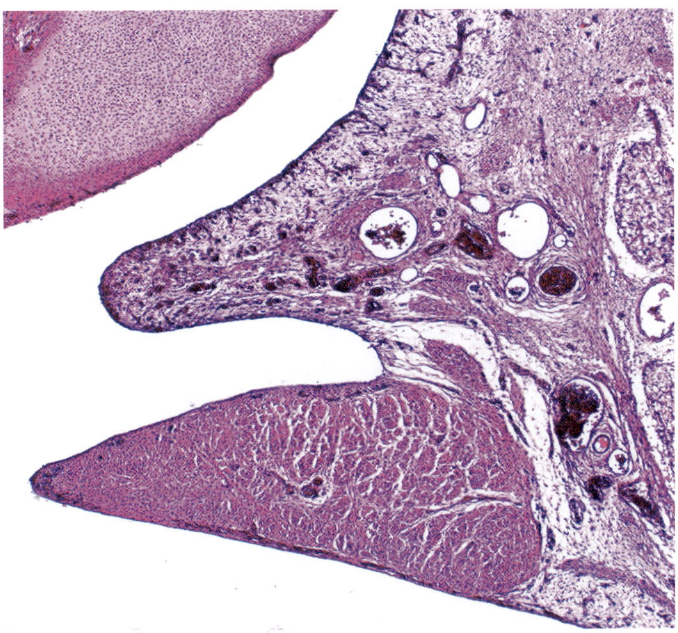

Fig. 13-26. Sagittal section of meniscus in a 170 mm fetus, showing collagenous fibers and blood vessels. The bundles of collagenous fibers are in general parallel to each other. A villus in the infrapatellar region projects into the joint cavity. The loose connective tissue comprising the subintima contains several blood vessels.

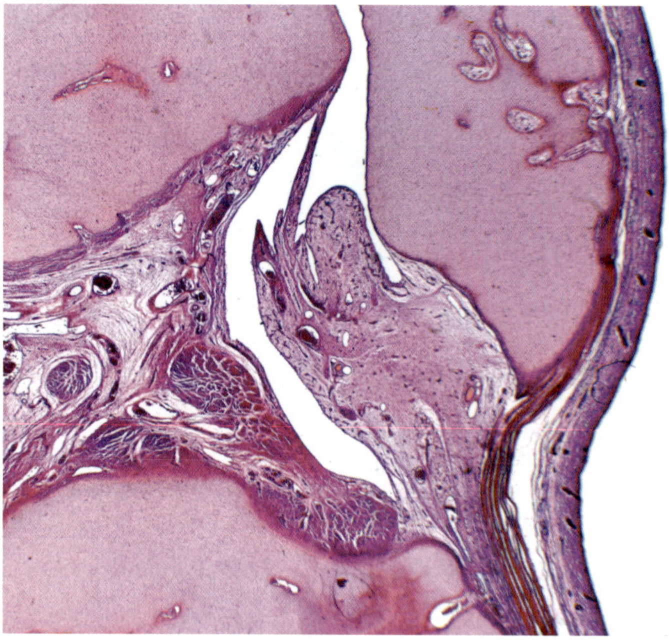

Fig. 13-27. Sagittal section through the knee joint from a 200 mm fetus to show the vascular synovial tissue. Lobules of fat are numerous in the infrapatellar region and in the popliteal fossa.

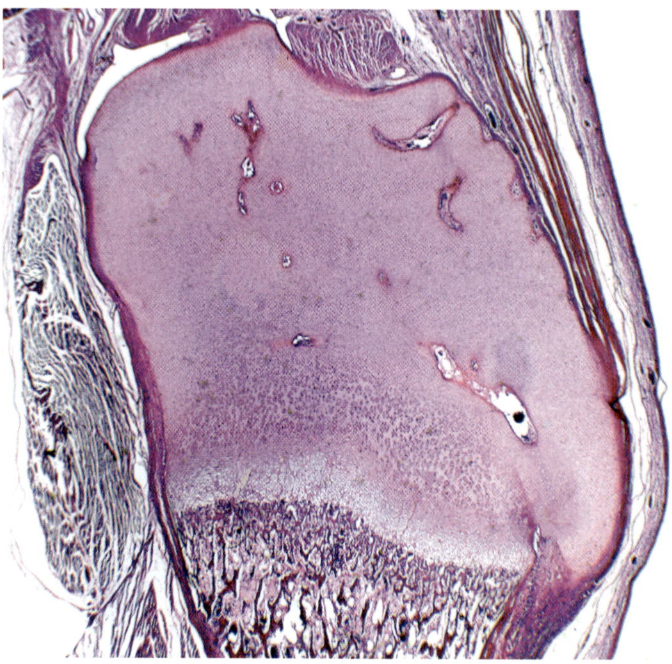

Fig. 13-28. Sagittal section through the knee joint in a 200 mm fetus to show endochondral bone formation. The endochondral bone formation of the tibia has reached the level of tibial tuberosity. The formation of the tibial tuberosity has progressed considerably. The columns of cartilage cells indicate that the growth plate is forming.

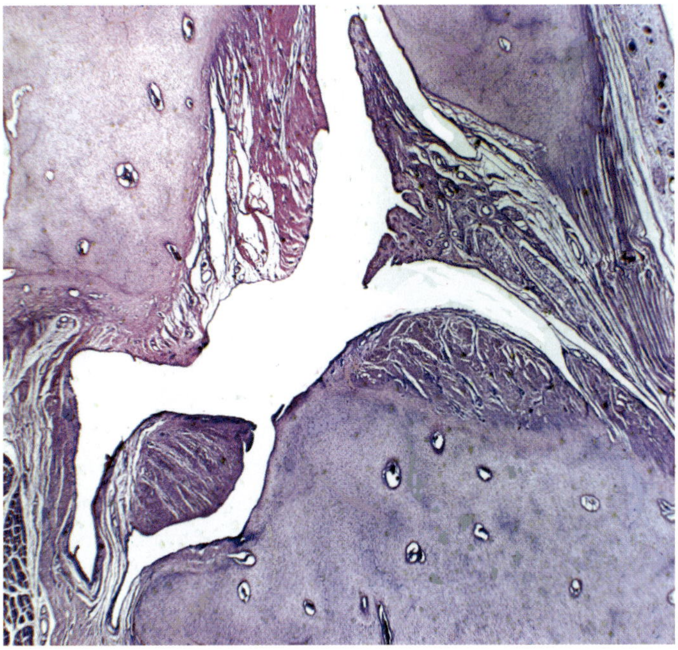

Fig. 13-29. Sagittal section through the knee joint in a 250 mm fetus to show vascular synovial tissue in the infrapatellar region. Several villi project into the cavity. The vascular network in the synovial membrane extends to the lining of the joint cavity.

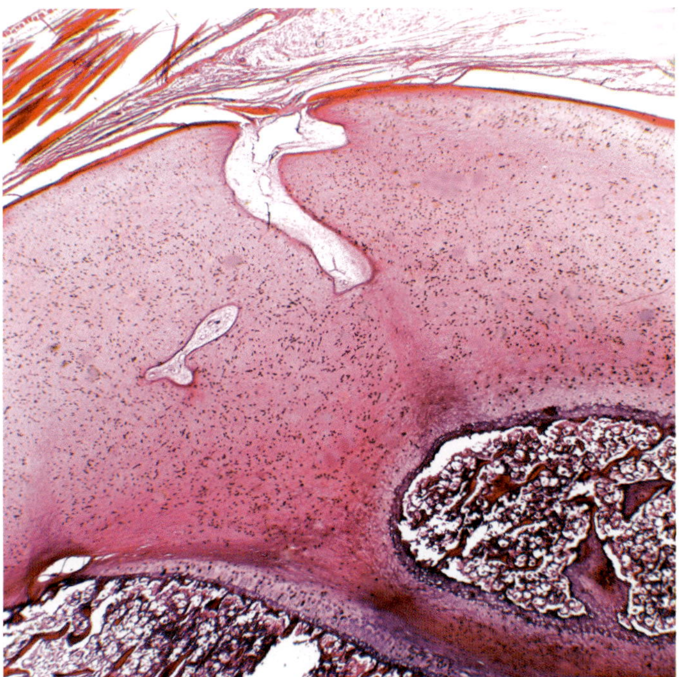

Fig. 13-30. Sagittal section through the part of the proximal tibia from a 300 mm fetus, showing the secondary ossification center of the proximal epiphysis. Endochondral bone formation has reached the level of tuberosity of the tibia.

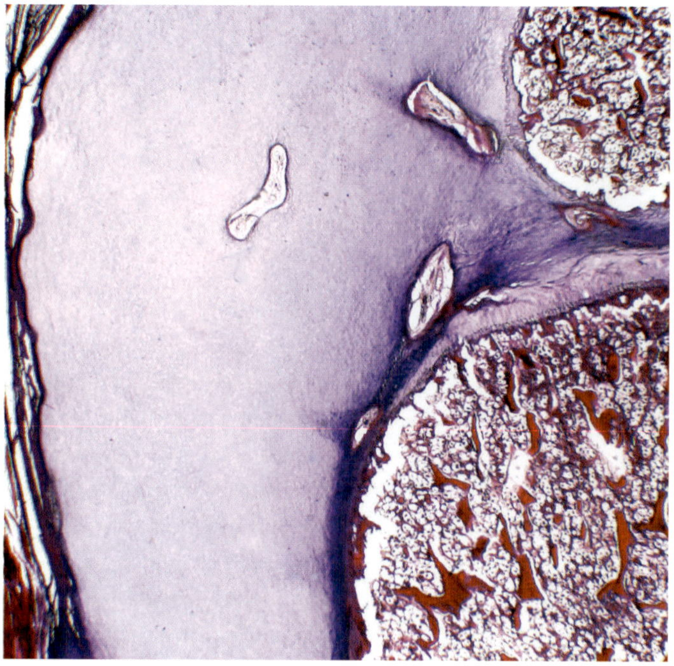

Fig. 13-31. Sagittal section through the part of the proximal tibia at one month of age, showing the secondary ossification center of the proximal epiphysis. The proximal growth plate has reached the level of tuberosity of the tibia.

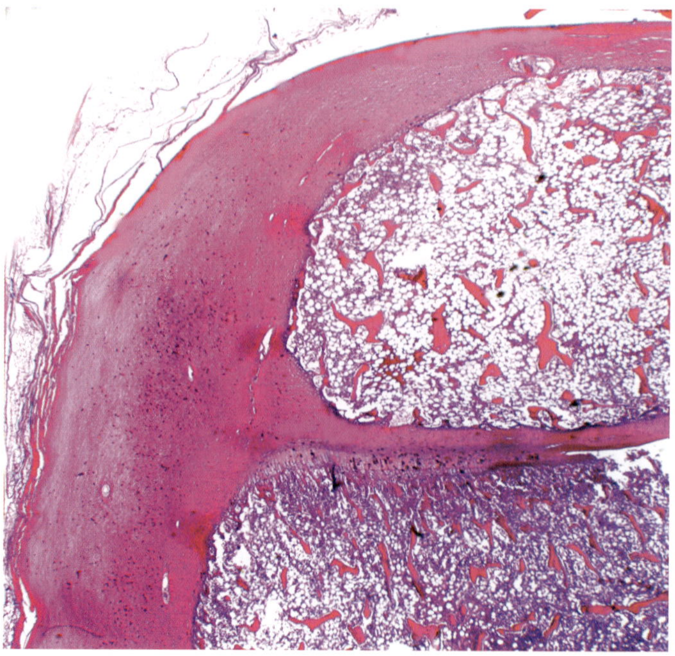

Fig. 13-32. Sagittal section through the part of the proximal tibia at one year after birth to show ossification along the metaphyseal side. Note many cartilage cells bordering the metaphyseal side of the bony center do not degenerate.

References

Chung JW: The prenatal development of the knee joint in Korean fetuses. *Chonnam Medical J* 8: 239-254, 1971.

Doskocil M: Formation of the femoropatellar part of the human knee joint. *Folia Morph* 33: 38-47, 1985.

Gray DJ, Gardner E: Prenatal development of the human knee and superior tibiofibular joints. *Am J Anat* 86: 235-287, 1950.

Haines RW: The early development of the femoro-tibial and tibio-fibular joints. *J Anat* 87: 192-206, 1953.

Kim BY, Joo KJ, Nam KI, Yoon JR: An ultrastructural study on the development of the knee joint in the human fetus. *Korean J Electron Microscopy* 30: 213-232, 2000.

McDermott LJ: Development of the human knee joint. *Arch Surg* 46: 705-719, 1943.

Moll J: The embryonic development of the human knee joint. *Act Neerl Morphol Nor Pathol* 6: 283-384, 1948.

O'Rahilly, R: The early prenatal development of the human knee joint. *J Anat* 85: 166-170, 1951.

The Development of the Ankle and Foot

Chapter 14

The appendicular skeleton consists of the pectoral and pelvic girdles, as well as the bones of the appendages themselves. In their basic plan of the structure, the arm and leg are closely comparable. Once it starts, the development of the appendicular skeleton progresses very rapidly. As it is universally agreed that the limb segment of human embryo follows the proximodistal origin of development, the embryological development of the tibia and fibula should precede that of the foot (Saunders, 1948). The skeletal elements of the thigh and leg appear as condensed mesenchyme before those of the foot. The femur begins to chondrify before the tibia, and the tibia before the elements of the foot. Chondrification of the tibia and fibula is already completed in the 23 mm embryo (Fig. 14-1). In the foot, chondrification begins in the metatarsal, slightly ahead of the tarsus. All elements of the foot except sesamoids usually begin to chondrify by the 21 and 25 mm embryos (Figs. 14-1 and 14-2). By the 35 mm fetus, general form of the skeletal elements in the talocrural and intertarsal joints resembles that of the adult (Fig. 14-5). Erosion of the bony collar by a periosteal bud is noted and the ossification center is first seen in the tibia from 30 mm on, and in the fibular from 35 mm on.

The ossification of the calcaneus and the talus begins during the fetal period. The calcaneus is the first tarsal bone to ossify. The periosteal bone formation is noted on the inferolateral aspect of the calcaneus by the 130 mm fetus (Fig. 14-23). In the 150 mm fetus, hypertrophied chondrocytes are first noted (Fig. 14-31). Endochondral ossification is first observed in the 180 and 200 mm fetuses (Figs. 14-32 and 14-33). The ossification center in the talus appears in the neck region in the 200 mm fetus (Fig. 14-33). The inconstant periosteal bone formation is followed by the appearence of the primary main center of talus in the 260 mm fetus (Figs. 14-35 and 14-36).

The distal phalanges are peculiar in their mode of ossification. In the 50 mm fetus, intramenbranous ossification of the tip of cartilaginous distal phalanx is first noted (Fig. 14-19). The tuberosity of the distal phalanx is formed by membranous bony trabeculae on the exterior of the subperiosteal cap in the 60 mm fetus (Fig. 14-20). By the 100 mm fetus, endochondral ossification is first observed in distal extremity of the distal phalanx. After the 150 mm fetus, endochondral and subperiosteal ossification proceed in only one direction, proximally (Fig. 14-21). These findings demonstrate that intramembranous ossification, calcification, and endochondral ossifiction start at the tip of the distal phalanx instead of at the center of the shaft, as is the case in other long bones. In each, the distal phalanx is followed by the metatarsal, proximal phalanx, and middle phalanx, in that order.

Hypertrophied cartilage cells are first noted in the metatarsus in the 50 mm fetus (Fig. 14-8). A primary bone collar of metatarsals is first seen in the 55 mm fetus (Fig. 14-24), and endochondral ossification in the 80 mm fetus (Fig. 14-27). As endochondral ossification proceeds proximally and distally, periosteal bone formation also proceeds longitudinally until about the 220 mm fetus (Fig. 14-28).

Talocalcaneal and calcaneonavicular fusions are noted in the 50 and 60 mm fetuses, respectively (Figs. 14-11 and 14-12). All fusions are cartilaginous. No accessory cartilages are found, but a bipartite medial cuneiform is seen in 80 mm fetus (Fig. 14-18).

The talus is the first of the tarsals to show vascular invasion. The cartilage canals are first present in the talus in the 80 mm fetus (Fig. 14-17), and are constantly present in the talus in the 100 mm fetus (Fig. 14-22). The cartilage canals are present in calcaneus in the 100 mm fetus (Fig. 14-22) and in all tarsus in the 200 mm fetus (Figs. 14-29, 14-30, and 14-33). The cartilage canals of the talus and calcaneus are identified as vascular channels arising from perichondrium surfaces. Superficial, intermediate, and deep canals in the talus and calcaneus are identified by the characteristics of cartilage cells. A number of cartilage canals are seen around the developing center of ossification in the talus and calcaneus (Fig. 14-33).

The medial and lateral cartilaginous sesamoids of interphalngeal joint of the great toe are observed in the 60 mm fetus (Fig. 14-25). The interphalangeal and metatarsophalangeal sesamoids of the great toe are found in the 130 mm fetus (Fig. 14-26). The findings on distribution of cartilaginous sesamoids are roughly similar to those reported for the adult.

The homogenous interzone and three-layered interzone in the talocrural and subtalar joints are present in the 23 mm embryo (Fig. 14-2) and 30 mm fetus (Fig. 14-3). Primitive joint cavities of the talocrural and intertarsal joints are present around the periphery of the joint in the 45 and 50 mm fetuses (Figs. 14-6 and 14-9) and are completed between 70 and 100 mm fetuses (Figs. 14-10, 14-13, and 14-22). A cleft appears in the lower ends of the tibia and fibula by the 35 mm (Fig. 14-4) and is separated from talocrural joint cavity by the thin cellular strand thereafter. After the 50 mm fetus, the tibiofibular cleft communicates with the talocrural joint cavity (Fig. 14-7).

The appearance of the fibrous capsule of the talocrural joint is followed by the completion of the skeletal elements in the joint, and fibrous capsule is observed as the condensation of collagenous fibers in the 60 mm fetus. The anterior portion of fibrous capsule is thin, and imperfectly developed near the talus, but posterior portion of the fibrous capsule consists of the thickened fibrous sheaths of the tibialis posterior and flexor hallucis longus tendons.

Ligaments are present as cellular condensations before cavities. From 30 mm fetus on, all other ligaments of the foot and ankle are present and become increasingly prominent by virtue of their collagenous fibers. A condensation for the long plantar ligament, the calcaneonavicular and calcaneocuboid parts of the bifurcated ligament, and deep transverse metartarsal ligament are noted in the 80 mm fetus (Fig. 14-10).

The tendon of the peroneus longus is differentiated in the 23 mm embryo (Fig. 14-2). The peroneus longus and other tendons have a sheath with a cavity in the 50 mm fetus (Fig. 14-8). By the 80 mm fetus, the tendon of the tibialis posterior is very cellular at its insertion into the navicular and gives off fibrous expansions (Fig. 14-14). The peroneus longus tendon crosses medially below the cuboid and is inserted into the lateral aspect of the first metatarsal bone (Fig. 14-16).

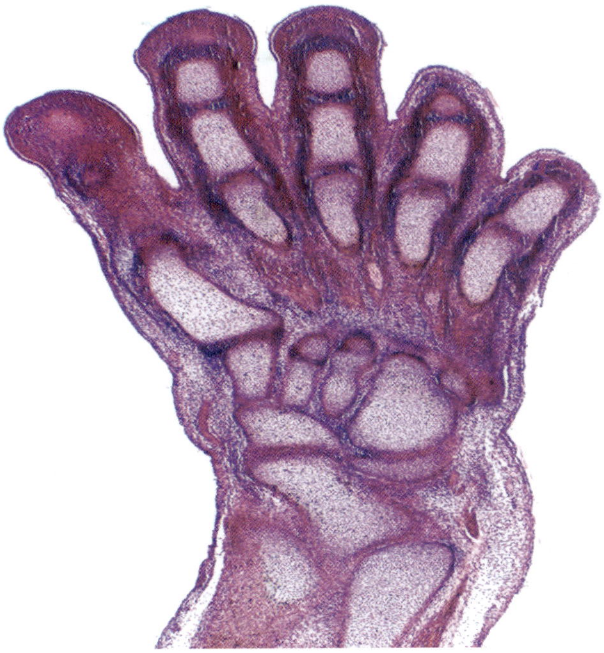

Fig. 14-1. Horizontal section through the part of the foot from a 23 mm embryo, showing chondrification of the lateral and medial malleoli, talus, calcaneus, navicular, cuboid, three cuneiforms, metatarsus, and proximal and distal phalanges. The peroneus longus tendon has a sheath with a cavity.

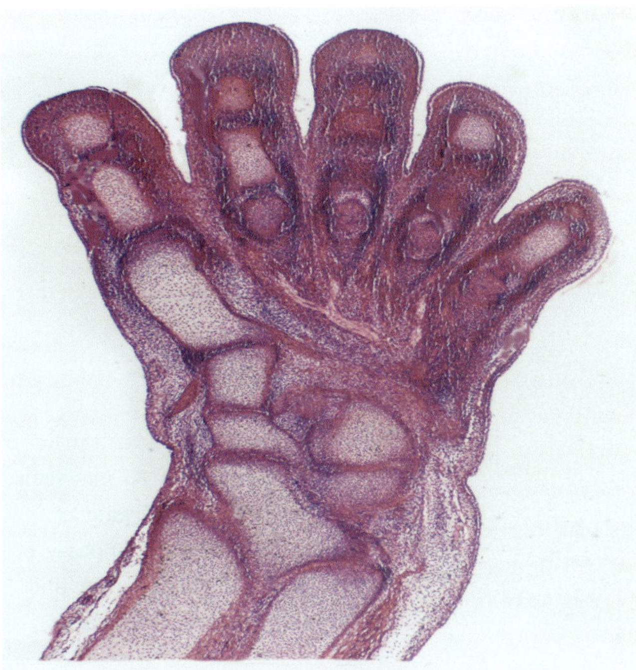

Fig. 14-2. Horizontal section through the part of the foot from a 23 mm embryo, showing chondrification of the tibia, fibula, tarsus, and metatarsus. The homogenous interzone can be seen in the ankle and other tarsal joints.

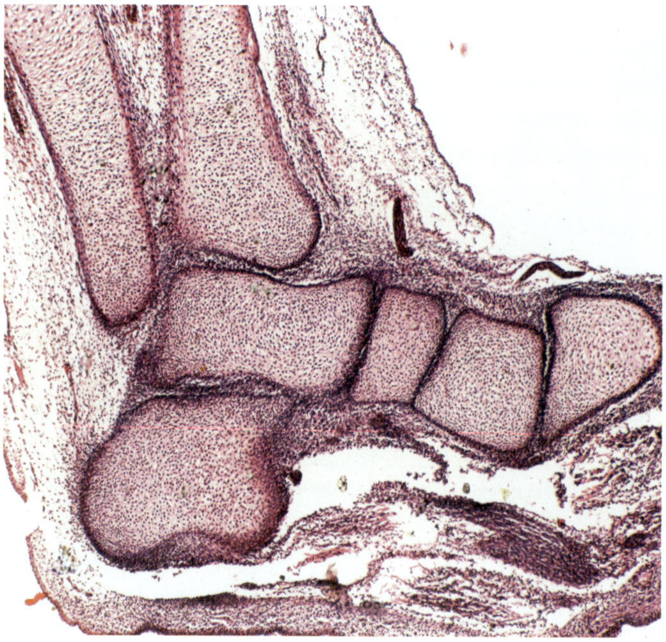

Fig. 14-3. Sagittal section of the foot from a 30 mm fetus, showing lateral and medial malleoli, talus, calcaneus, navicular, and tibialis anterior tendon. Chondrification of the tibia and fibula are copmleted. The ankle joint has developed into a three-layered interzone.

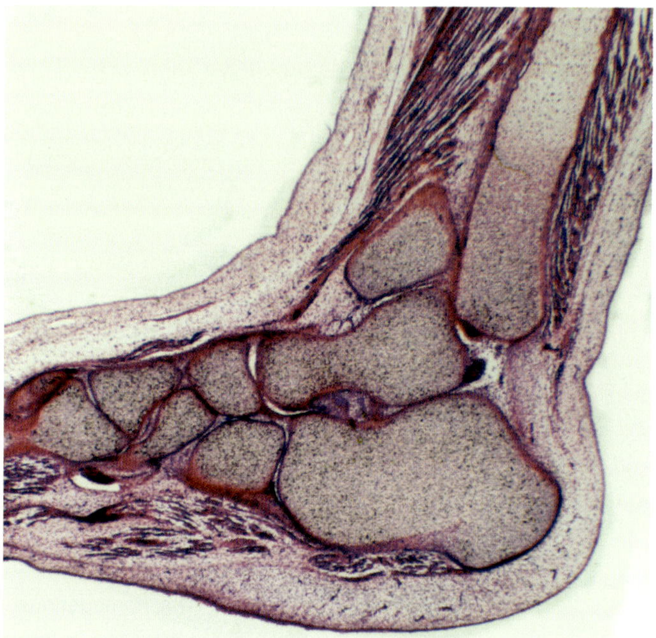

Fig. 14-4. Horizontal section of the foot from a 35 mm fetus, showing the beginning of cavitation at the periphery of talocrural, talonavicular, and calcaneocuboid interzones.

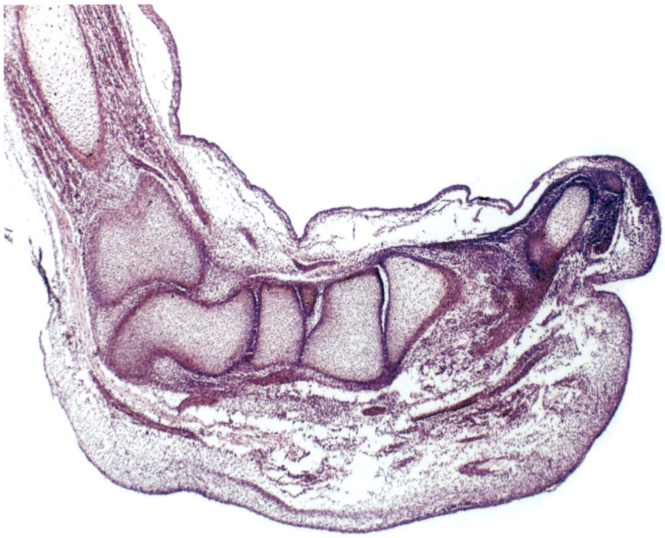

Fig. 14-5. Horizontal section through the part of the foot from a 35 mm fetus to show bipartite medial cuneiform. Cavitaton at the periphery of the interzone between the first metatarsal and medial cuneiform bones.

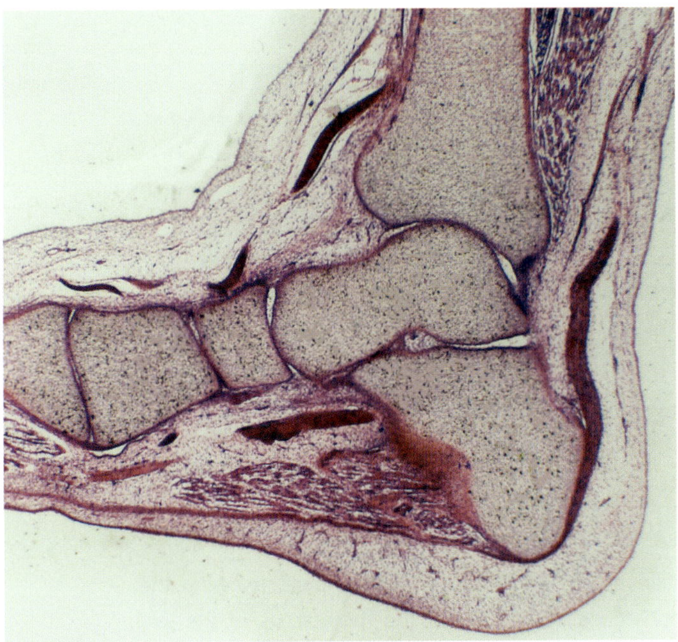

Fig. 14-6. Sagittal section through part of the foot from a 45 mm fetus to show the beginning of cavitation of the talocrural, talonavicular, and subtalar joints. The tibialis anterior tendon, tendo calcaneus and flexor digitorum longus tendon are seen. The tendo calcaneus inserts in the fibrous perichondrium of the posterior part of the calcaneus.

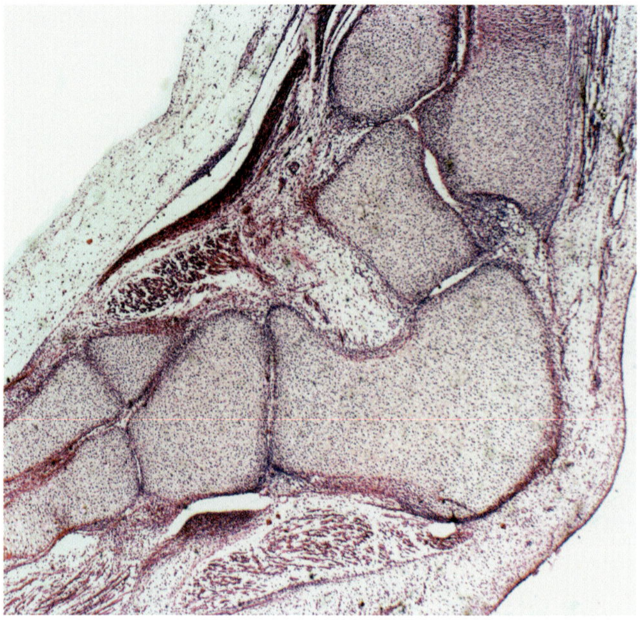

Fig. 14-7. Sagittal section of the foot from a 50 mm fetus to show the cavity of the talocrural and subtalar joints. The tibiofibular cleft communicates with the talocrural joint cavity. The tibialis anterior tendon is seen.

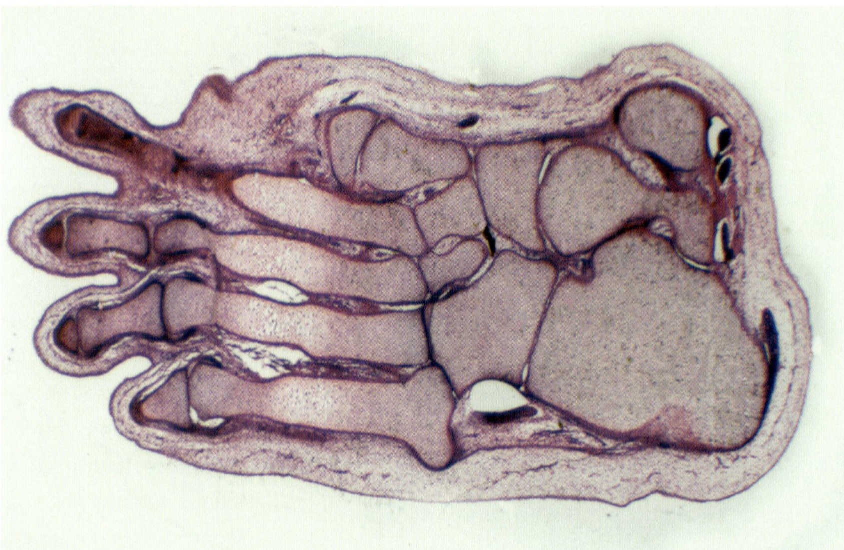

Fig. 14-8. Horizontal section of the foot from a 50 mm fetus, showing the bone collar and hypertrophied cartilage cells of the metatarsus of the 2nd, 3rd, 4th, and 5th toes. Note the cavitation in the synovial sheath on the tibialis posterior, flexor diditorum longus, and flexor hallucis longus. The peroneus longus tendon and cavity of its sheath are observed.

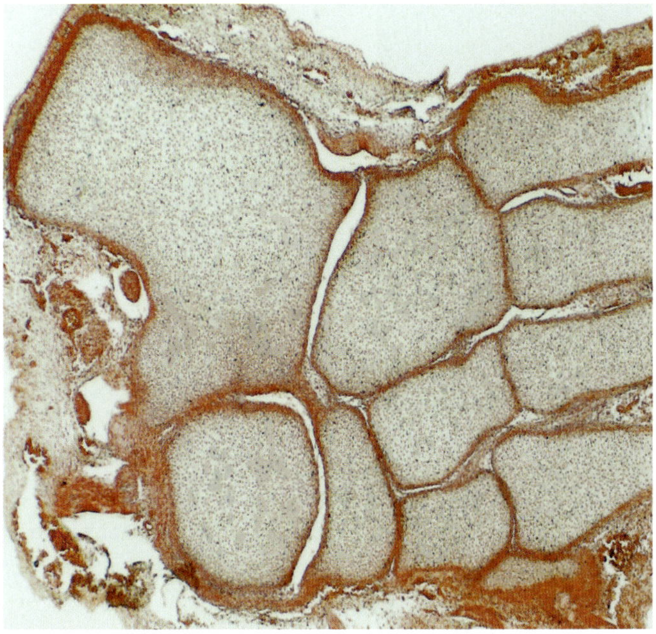

Fig. 14-9. Horizontal section of the foot from a 60 mm fetus to show the cavity in talocalcaneonavicular and calcaneocuboid joints.

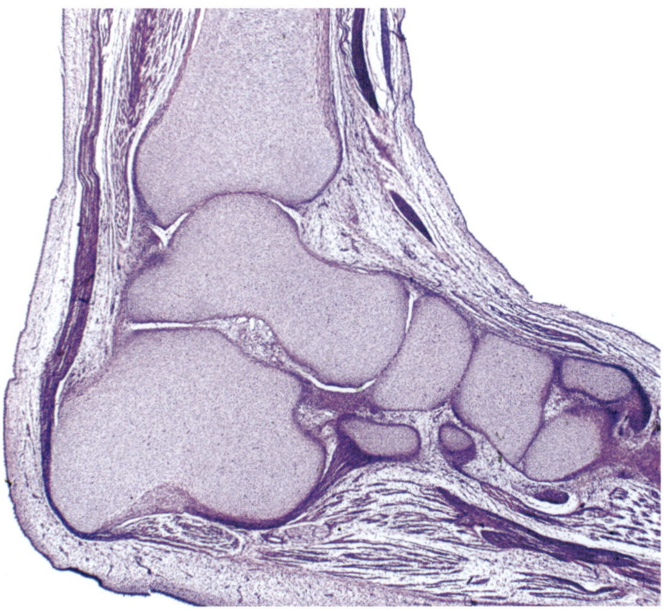

Fig. 14-10. Sagittal section of the foot from a 60 mm fetus, showing tendons of the tibialis anterior and triceps surae. The joint cavities are present in the talocrural, subtalar, and talocalcaneonavicular joints. The calcaneal tendon inserts in the perichodrium of the posterior surface of the calcaneus. The bifurcated calcaneonavicular and calcaneocuboid ligaments are seen.

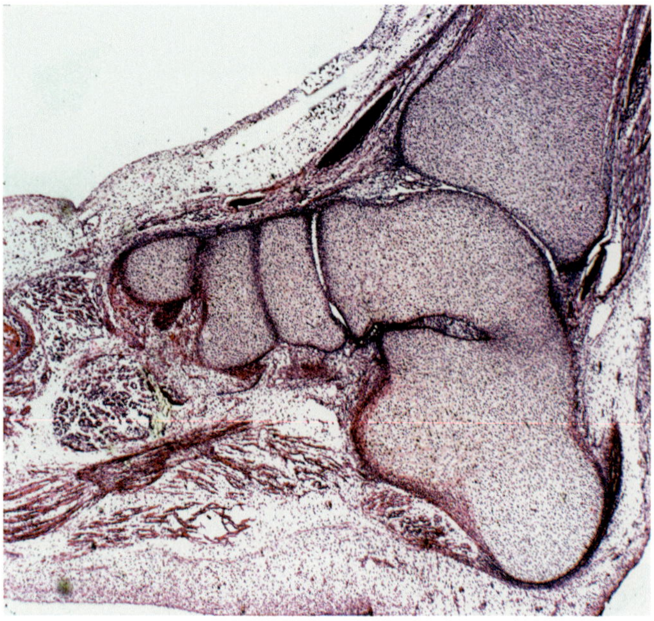

Fig. 14-11. Sagittal section of the foot in a 50 mm fetus, showing talocalcaneal fusion in the region of the sustentaculum tali.

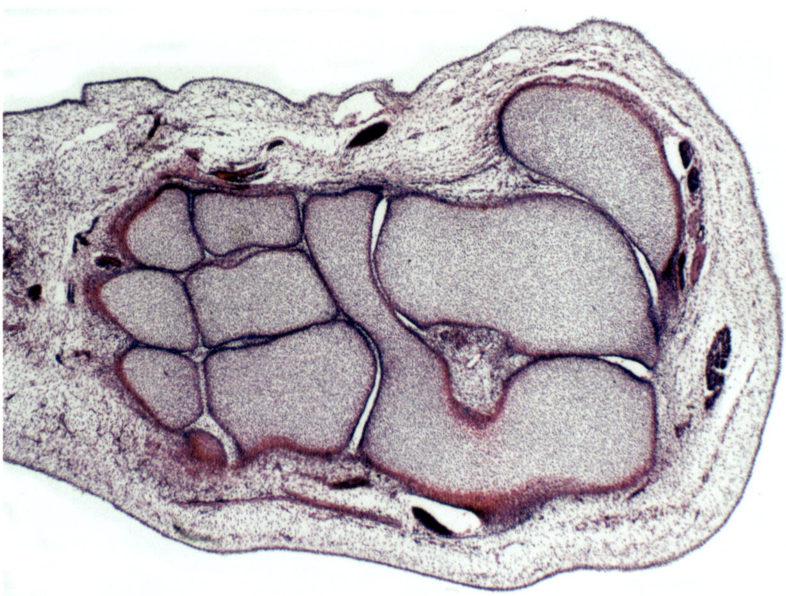

Fig. 14-12. Horizontal section of the foot from a 60 mm fetus, showing peripheral cavitation with the still-fused axial portion of the interzone in most of the ankle joint. Note the cartilaginous fusion between the calcaneus and navicular.

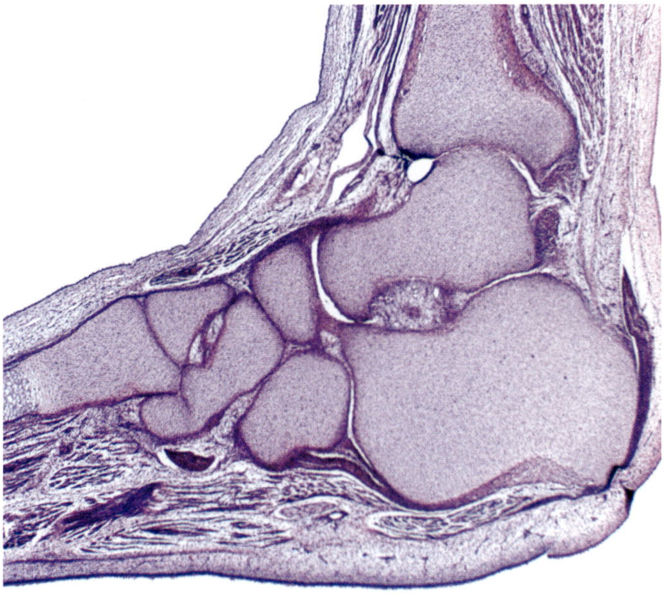

Fig. 14-13. Sagittal section of the foot from a 60 mm fetus, showing cavities in the talocalcaneonavicular and calcaneocuboid joints. Note the long and short plantar ligaments.

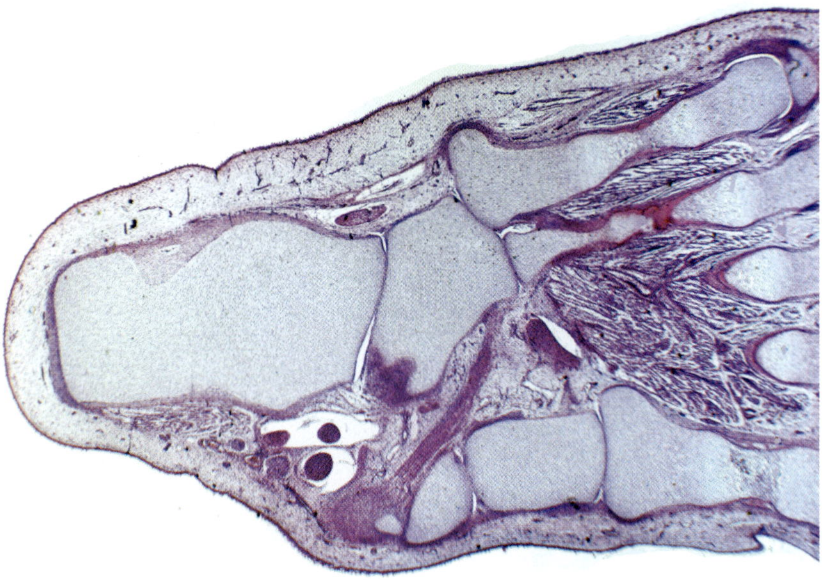

Fig. 14-14. Horizontal section of the foot from a 80 mm fetus, showing the calcaneus and cuboid above, and the navicular and medial cuneiform below. Note the distal prolongation of the tibialis posterior insertion.

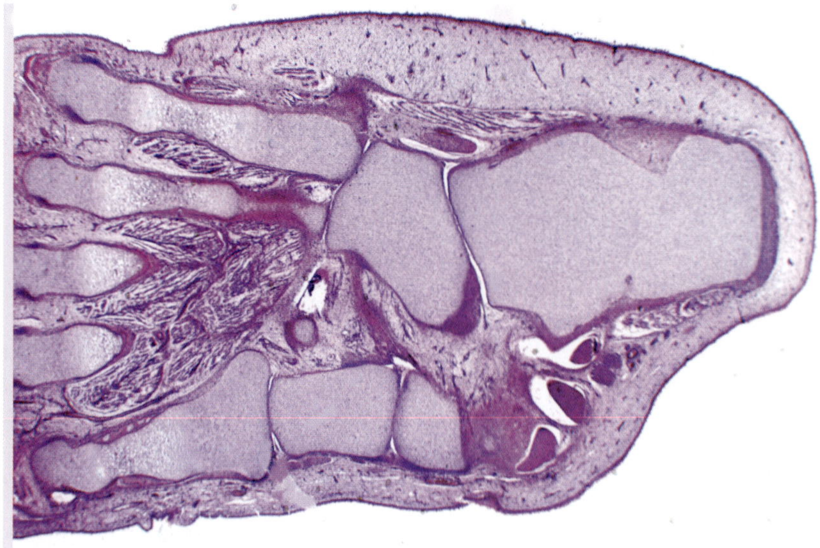

Fig. 14-15. Horizontal section of the foot from a 80 mm fetus, showing calcification of the hypertrophied cartilage in the fourth and fifth metatarsal bones. A cartilage canal is found in the calcaneus. The peroneus longus and tibialis posterior tendons have a sheath with a cavity.

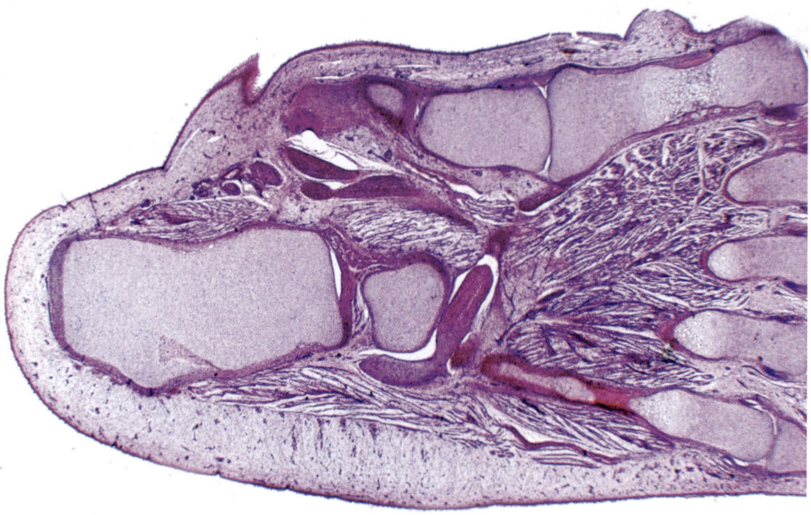

Fig. 14-16. Horizontal section of the foot from a 80 mm fetus, showing the peroneus longus tendon turning medially below the cuboid. Its insertion is mainly into the first metatarsal bone.

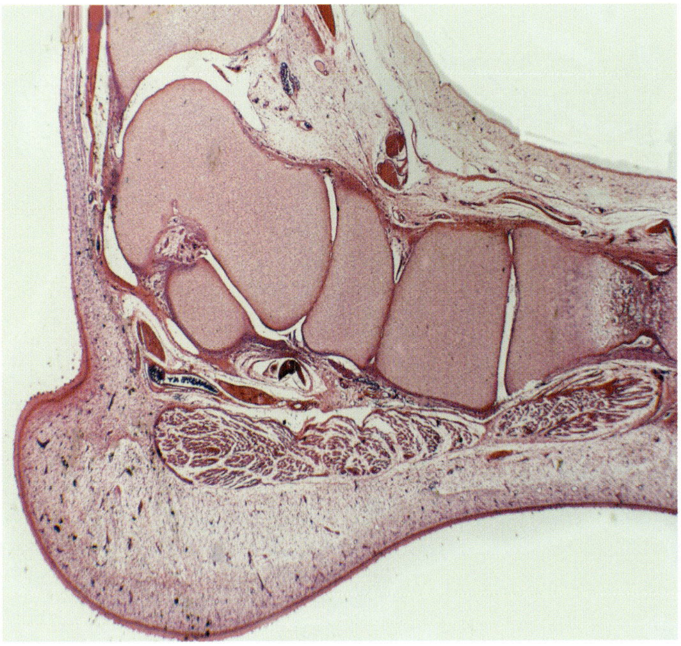

Fig. 14-17. Sagittal section from a 80 mm fetus to show the definitive talocrural, subtalar, and intertarsal joints. Initial appearance of the cartilage canal in the talus is seen. The first metatarsal has a bone collar which is beginning to erode.

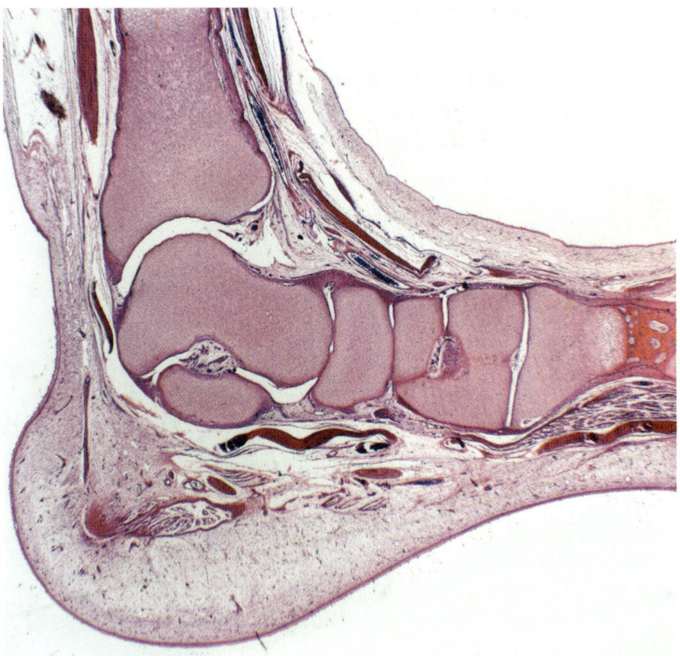

Fig. 14-18. Sagittal section through part of the foot from a 80 mm fetus, showing a bipartite medial cuneiform.

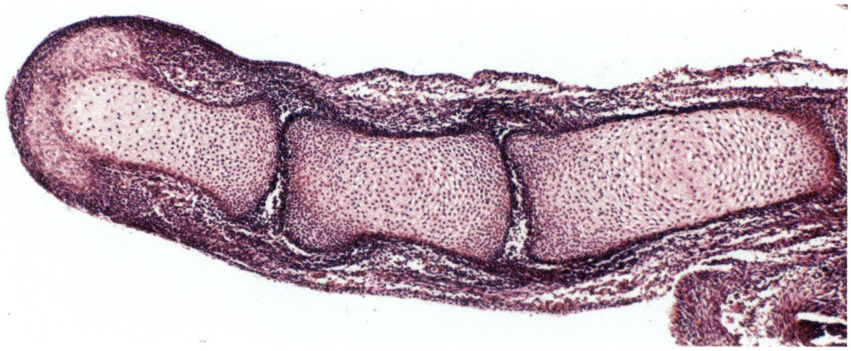

Fig. 14-19. Sagittal section from a 50 mm fetus, showing early membranous ossification at the tip of a distal phalanx of the great toe.

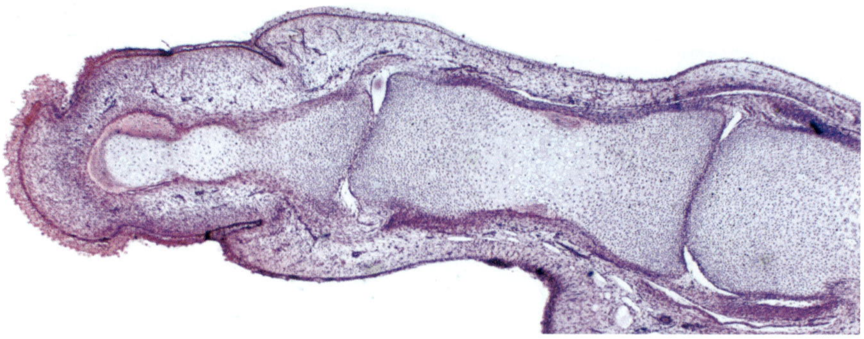

Fig. 14-20. Sagittal section from a 60 mm fetus, showing membranous ossification at the tip of the distal phalanx. A shell of subperiosteal bone is deposited, which resembles a thimble over the cartilaginous phalanx.

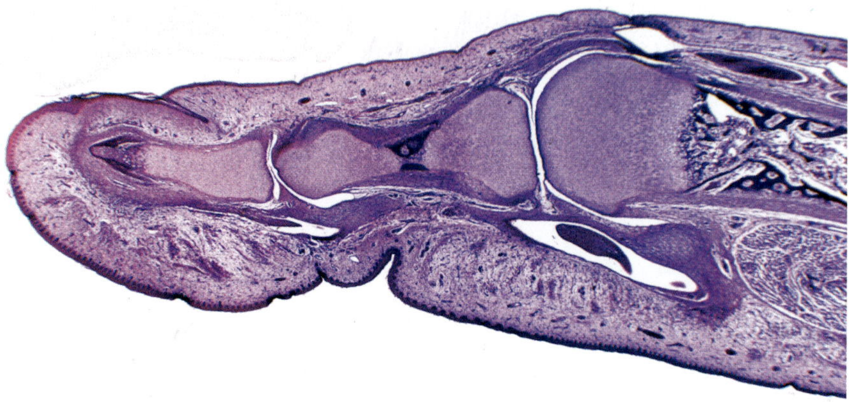

Fig. 14-21. Sagittal section from a 150 mm fetus, showing membranous ossification at the tip of the distal phalanx. Periosteal bone extends proximally beyond the level of endochondral ossification.

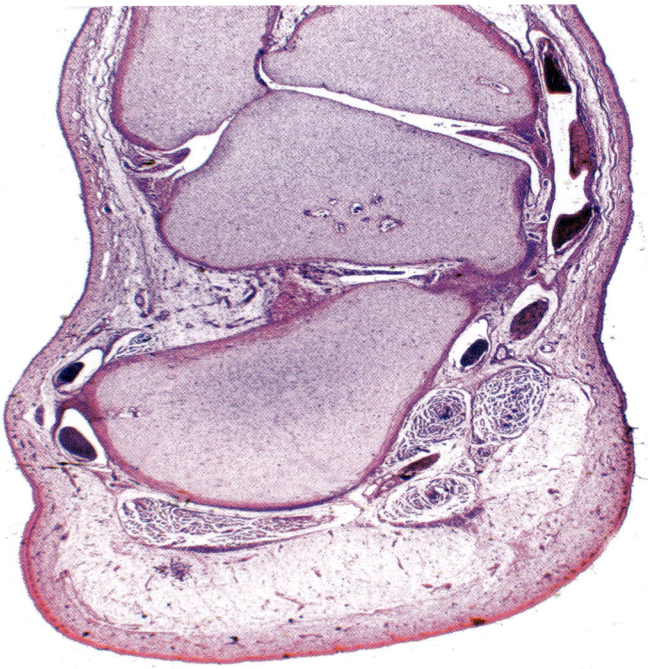

Fig. 14-22. Frontal section of the foot from a 100 mm fetus to show the sinus tarsi. Cartilage canals in the tibia, talus and calcaneus are seen. Vascular synovial folds are present in the ankle joint.

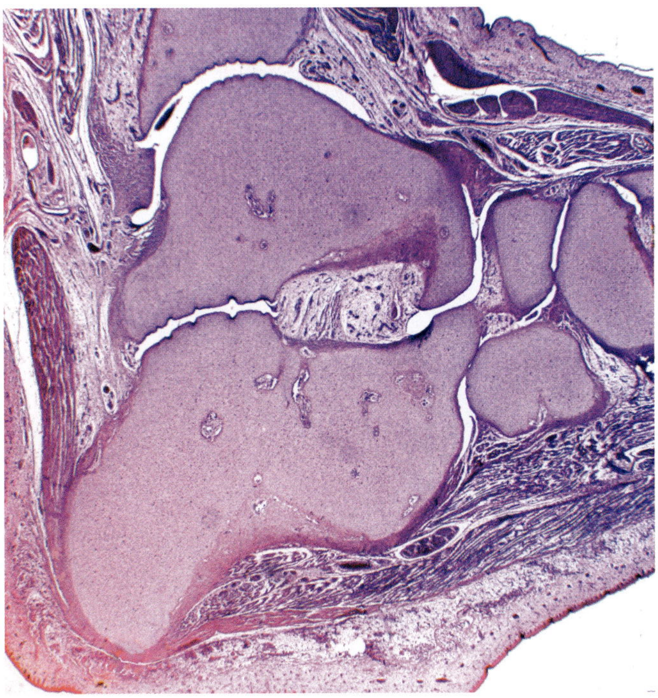

Fig. 14-23. Sagittal section of the foot in a 110 mm fetus, showing the periosteal bone at the postero-inferolateral aspect of the calcaneus. The cartilage canals in the talus, calcaneus, and cuboid are observed. Note the entrance of the vessels from the tarsal canal.

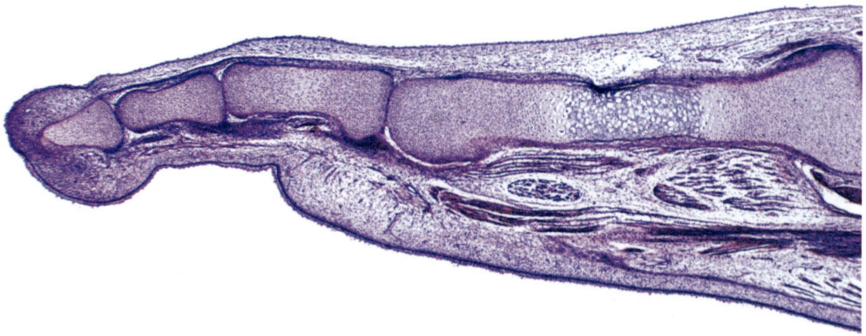

Fig. 14-24. Sagittal section of the finger from a 55 mm fetus to show subperiosteal bone formation of the metatarsal bone. Note the proximal and middle phalanges that resemble the adult element in shape.

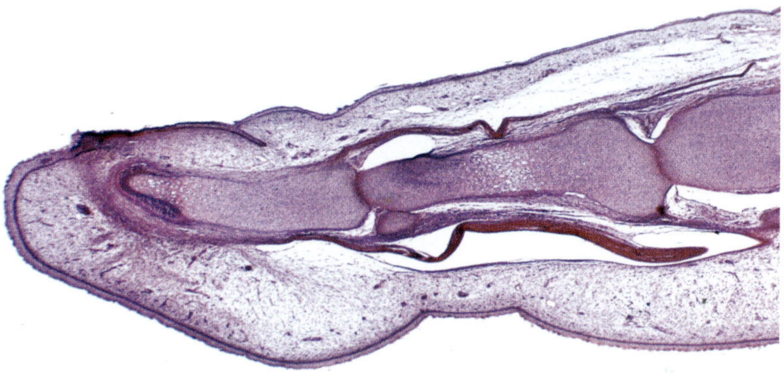

Fig. 14-25. Sagittal section of the great toe in a 60 mm fetus to show interphalangeal sesamoid. Membranous bone formation at the tip is noted.

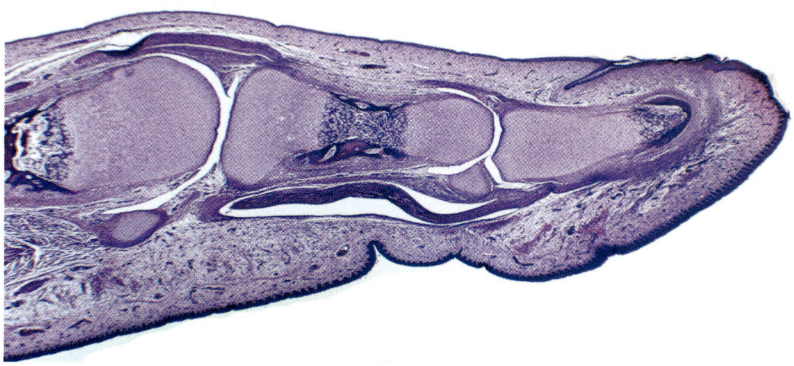

Fig. 14-26. Sagittal section of the great toe from a 130 mm fetus to show interphalangeal and metatarsophalangeal sesamoids of the great toe. Endochondral ossification of phalanges and metatarsus of the great toe is noted. Subperiosteal bone of the proximal phalanx and metatarsus extends proximally and distally beyond the level of endochondral ossification.

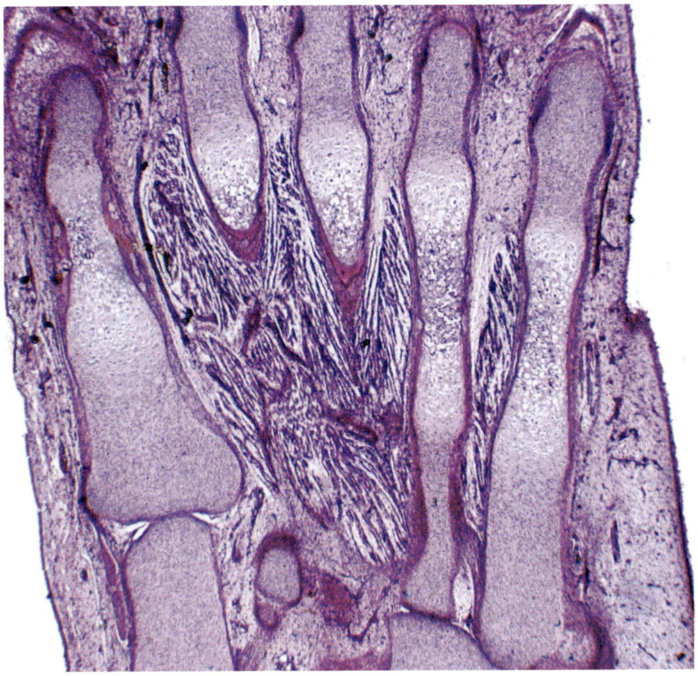

Fig. 14-27. Sagittal section of the foot from a 80 mm fetus, showing the extent of periosteal-bone formation in the metatarsal bones. The periosteal bone extends into the level of endochondral ossification.

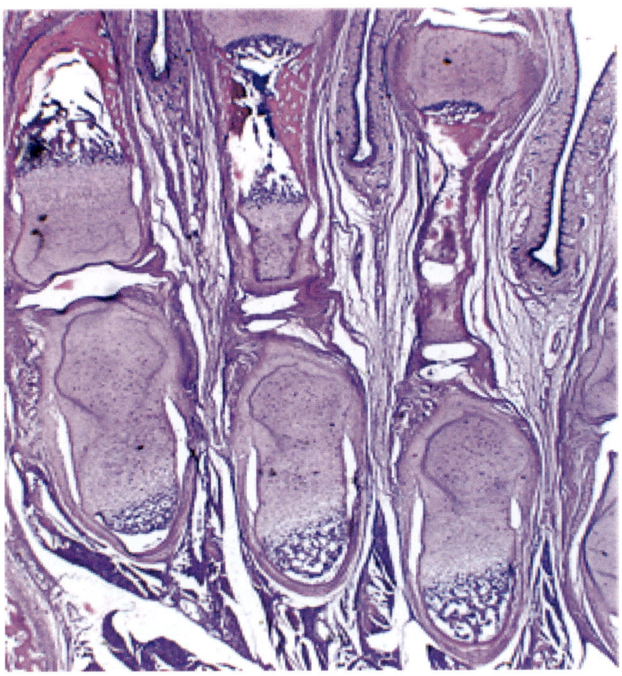

Fig. 14-28. Sagittal section of the foot from a 220 mm fetus, showing endochondral ossification of the phalanges and the metatarsal bones. From left to right: proximal phalanges of the second, third, and fourth toes, showing endochondral trabeculae with a periosteally formed shell.

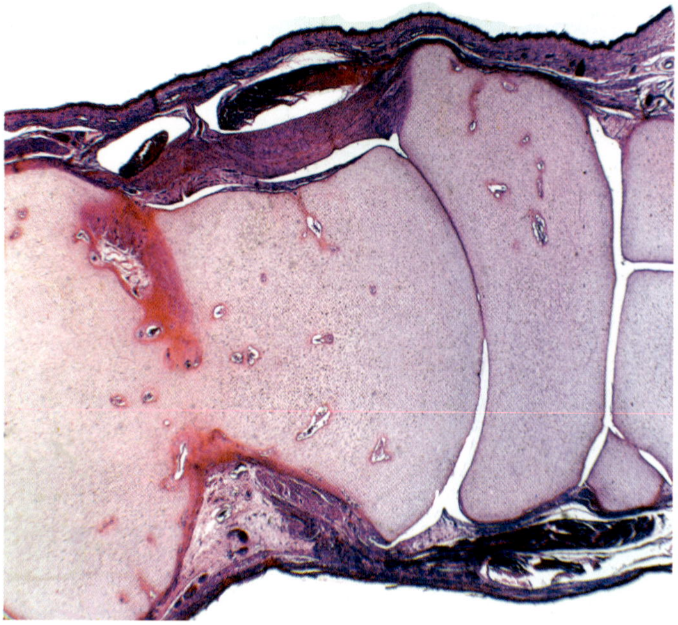

Fig. 14-29. Sagittal section of the foot from a 130 mm fetus to show cartilage canals in the talus and navicular. Note the tibialis posterior tendon, which joins the plantar calcaneonavicular ligament.

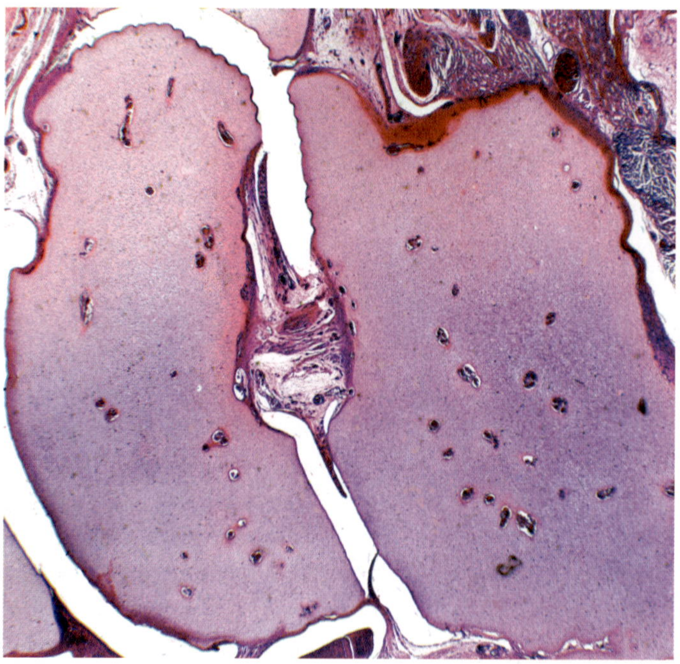

Fig. 14-30. Sagittal section of foot in a 160 mm fetus to show the cartilage canals in the talus and calcaneus. Note the entrance of the vessels from the tarsal canal.

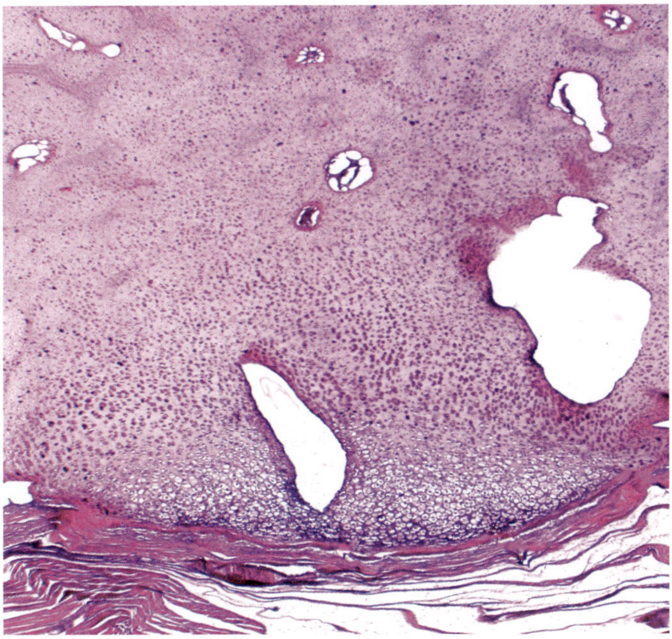

Fig. 14-31. Horizontal section of the calcaneus in a 150 mm fetus, showing a thin layer of subperiosteal bone on the inferolateral aspect of the calcaneus. The cartilage cells at the site of the main center of ossification are at the stage of hypertrophy. A number of cartilage canals form arcades around the center.

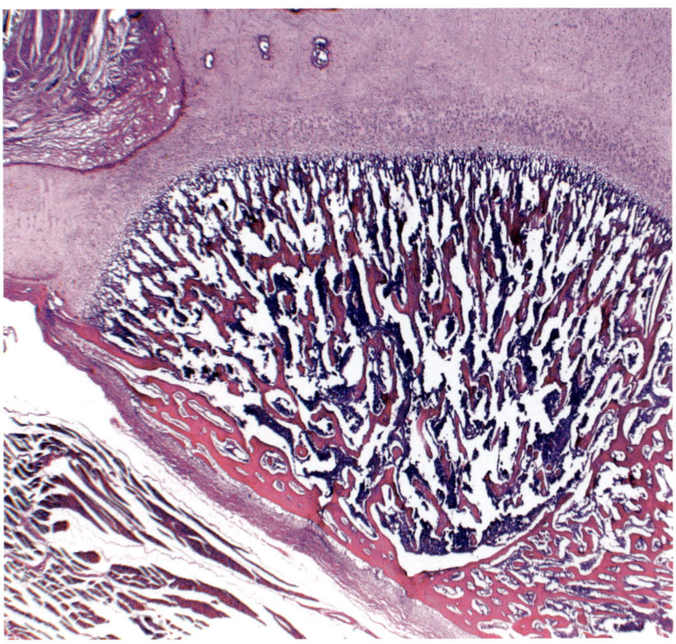

Fig. 14-32. Horizontal section of a 180 mm fetus to show endochondral ossification in the calcaneus. A single oval center of ossification merges with the parachondral center.

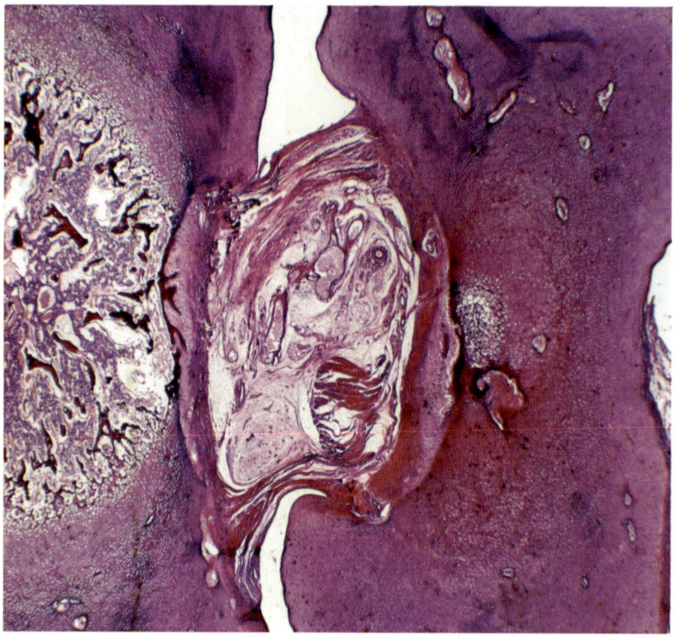

Fig. 14-33. Horizontal section through part of the talus and calcaneus in the 200 mm fetus, showing endochondral ossification in the calcaneus. Note the initial osteogenesis of the talus and its association with cartilage canals.

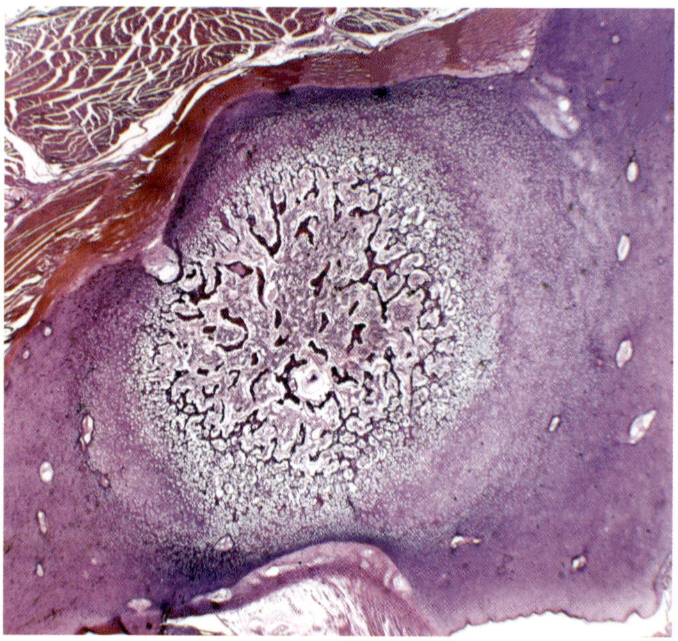

Fig. 14-34. Horizontal section of the talus in a 260 mm fetus to show endochondral trabeculae in the calcaneus. Endochondral ossification and its association with cartilage canals are seen in the calcaneus.

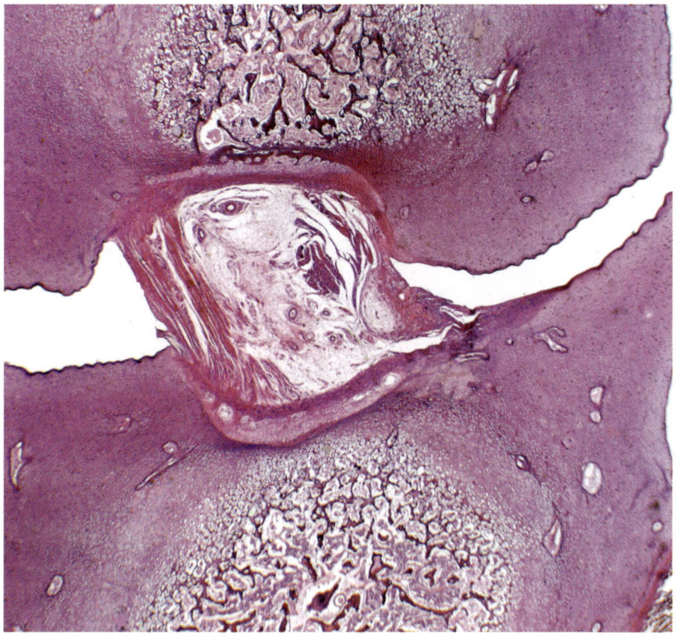

Fig. 14-35. Horizontal section through part of the talus and calcaneus in a 260 mm fetus, showing endochondral ossification in the talus and calcaneus. The vascular synovial fold in the sinus tarsi is seen.

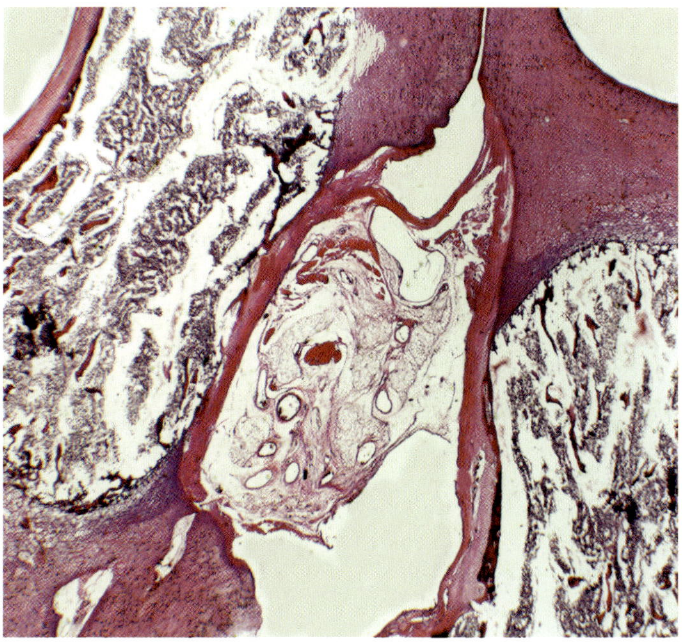

Fig. 14-36. Horizontal section through part of the talus and calcaneus in the 300 mm fetus, showing lobules of the fat, irregularly arranged connective tissue, and talocalcaneal interosseous ligament of sinus tarsi. Note the endochondral ossification in the talus and calcaneus.

References

Agrawal P, Atre PR, Kulkarni DS: The role of cartilage canals in the ossification of the talus. *Acta Anat* 119: 238-140, 1984.

Bae CS: The development of human talocrural and intertarsal joints during the fetal period. *The Korean J Anat* 12: 41-54, 1979.

Gardner E, Gray DJ, O'Rahilly R: The prenatal development of the skeleton and joints of the human foot. *J Bone Joint Surg* 41: 847-879, 1959.

Kawashima T, Uhthoff HK: Prenatal development around the sustentaculum tali and its relation to talocalcaneal coalition. *J Pediatr Orthop* 10: 238-243, 1990.

O'Rahilly R, Gardner E, Gray DJ: The skeletal development of the foot. *Clin Orthop* 16: 7-14, 1960.

Saunders JW: The proximo-distal sequence of origin of the parts of the chick wing and the role of the ectoderm. *J Exp Zool* 108: 363-404, 1948.

Index

P

R

S

T

V

Z